# The Tree of Happiness Mental Disorders

### By Cynthia Stevison

## Seven Practical Steps for Educating, Empowering, and Encouraging Others with Mental Illness

# Dedications:

For my family.
For the best supportive partner and friend.
For my children, may you dream big and find your purpose.
And for my tribe of friends.
If you are reading this book,
then chances are you are part of that tribe.
Thank you for sharing the belief that recovery is possible.

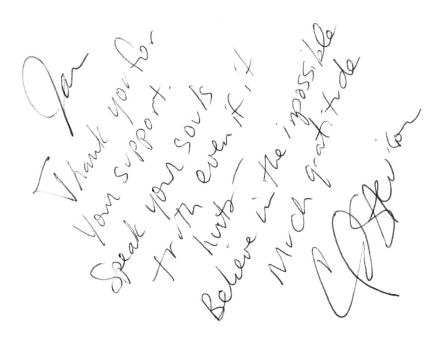

Edited by Deanna Mavis

# Acknowledgements of Praise:

"Listen. Why is that so hard? We, as human beings, are all connected. We have the same blood, the same Creator, but gigantically different stories, monumentally different struggles. We need to hear each others' stories. It is what connects us as fellow travelers on this human journey. Cynthia Stevison exposes her soul, courageously telling us her story. It is a story we need to hear and, more significantly, understand. But how can we understand? Most of us can never say, "I get it," because we have no idea how to walk in the shoes of persons with mental illness. But we can listen. We can help, not fix, but help. Choose to listen. Choose to notice. Choose to be present. Choose to connect in helpful ways. Be courageous, like Cynthia."

**Rev. Jeni Markham Clewell**

"I met Cindy at a gathering some two years ago. Little did I know as we spoke that fateful night, the profound sacred journey Cindy had already endured and where her road had always been leading her. *The Tree of Happiness* is deeply personal, raw retrieval of a family's trans-generational healing. It is a courageous study of the stigma of mental illness, a witnessing of our fear of the unknown, in the face of our sense of helplessness. Cindy tells an unfortunately, not uncommon, real story of her families surviving the multilevel facets of mental illness. Her quest to bring light to the miss handling of mental illness and the real steps and tools for recovery is disturbing, enlightening and inspiring.

Cindy is courageous, insightful, raw, wounded and wise as she takes us through the shadowy dark forest of mental illness and into the fresh sunlight of recovery and peace.

Thank you Cindy for your strength of character and perseverance in the face of your inner demons to revel the road to victory. I am better for having read your moving story of hope and recovery. Thank you for letting me see the view from your Tree of Happiness."

**Karen "Karuna" Harris, Karuna Personal Development**

"I have been a Licensed Clinical Social worker for 30 years and, in that capacity, have worked primarily in the provision of services to individuals and families experiencing and effected by mental illness and chemical dependency. Much of that time was spent working on specialized units or in private practice.

Part of the struggle in working with these population is the difficulty in getting individuals to re-focus their fears in healthy channels of self-responsibility and acceptance. The other is the advocacy necessary to the improve the overall understanding of these illnesses in ways that will contribute improved programs and treatment.

I first met Cynthia in 2003, long before her personal issues and insight lead her to the motivation that seeded the Tree of Happiness. I knew when I met her that her visions would become something bigger than even she knew. She is a wise woman, who has affected so many with her voracious desire to understand all things in ways that far exceed expectations.

There are many books, written by vast numbers of novice professionals, which claim to punctuate the need for improved understanding of mental health and addiction issues. Too often these are disappointing pieces of rhetoric, which plagiarize the philosophies rendered by professional counselors and therapists. This book is not the same!

Cynthia has opened up her heart in a brutally honest expose of her own journey. She has not only shared her humbling experiences, but has been generous enough to offer her own tools for the purpose of recovery.

I love this book and the way the very layman qualities reflected by Cynthia's writing styles allows people to fall into the comfort of being safe and normal.

I recommend it to everyone and am proud that the author has shared her life, her love and her words with so many!"

**Tama Cochran, LCSW**

## Disclaimers:

This book contains information that is intended to help the readers be better informed consumers about mental health issues. It is presented as general advice on health care. Always consult your therapist or psychiatrist for your individual needs.

Parts of my family do not want this story told. Names and characteristics have been changed so no harm may befall those still fighting mental illness. Some people fear discrimination if this story is written. This is not my intention. Rather, it is a story of recovery offering help and hope for those suffering. We must know that we can survive and pursue our purpose.

# Dear Reader,

I wrote this book to help you. Whether you are suffering from mental illness or know someone who is.

I hope you will read and reread "Part 2 – The Recovery Toolkit," as this was the key to my success and my healing. I hope it will be the same for you. Those seven steps can help you work through any problem.

In addition, I'm included journaling questions periodically throughout the book. They are meant for you to use in a therapeutic setting. Writing everything down can help. It will get you thinking.

I also share with you my story in hopes that you can relate. That you are inspired to improve and transform. That you will find hope and comfort.

Recovery is possible.


Sending hope and healing,

Cynthia Stevison

# Contents

Introduction..............................................................11
**Part 1 – The Struggle..........................................13**
Safe Cell................................................................15
Family Ties........................................................... 19
The Journey...........................................................31
Mental Evaluation................................................41
Surviving the 3 D's:
     Divorce.........................................................53
     Death............................................................57
     Disease........................................................ 63
Discharge............................................................ 69
Back to the Workforce......................................... 79
**Part 2 – The Recovery Toolkit...........................83**
The Plan: *Seven Practical Steps for Improving Your Health and Wellness*................................................ 85
Step One: *Recognition – Name the Disorder*...... 87
Step Two: *Expansion – Become an Architect of Your Own Destiny*.............................................. 95
Step Three: *Wellness Plan – Manage Crises*........99
Step Four: *Implementation – Put Your Plan into Action*....... 103
Step Five: *Evaluation – Determine the Benefits*................... 105
Step Six: *Education – Educate Yourself and Others*............ 109
Step Seven: *Empowerment – Achieve a Greater Sense of Confidence*................................................ 115
Photographs........................................................ 124
**Part 3 – The Healing.........................................131**
Ending the Silence............................................... 133
Accepting............................................................ 137
Following the Plan............................................... 139
**Part 4 – The Impact...........................................141**
Contributing........................................................ 143
Networking.......................................................... 147
Gratitude............................................................. 151
Conclusion – Don't Give Up................................ 157
Afterward............................................................ 161
Sources and Notes............................................... 162

# Introduction: *The Tree of Happiness*

Mental illness can strike anyone. It knows no age limits, economic status, race, creed, or color. We all suffer pain in different ways. Losing control of one's mind can be incredibly scary. Imagine being locked in a cell, restrained, and stripped of all humanity. Imagine no access to food or water, no human contact and being left to urinate and defecate where you sleep. This abuse is shocking but often true. Many Americans face these conditions each day believing it could be their last. There is a mental health crisis in our country and we must find liberation.

The Tree of Happiness begins with suffering and concludes with enlightenment. The story offers hope and healing to those willing to accept it and climb into their true potential. Slow, steady effort is the key to healing.

Journaling questions are included for you, the reader, to answer about yourself. They can help anyone, regardless if you have a mental illness or have a loved one who does.

The National Alliance on Mental Illness (Nami.org) is the source for most of the information and statistics is in this book, unless otherwise noted.

# Part 1 – The Struggle

## Safe Cell

I'm in a safe cell in the county jail. The officers want to prevent me from injuring myself, but more importantly, the other inmates. They keep constant watch over me in this dark concrete room. There are no fixtures, no bed, no toilet, no sink.

Just me, lying on the floor, naked.

This unsanitary environment is inhumane, with only a metal hole in the middle of the concrete room. I am alone, isolated and delusional. But I'm not afraid, and I'm not in pain.

In here, I am safe.

My name is Peter, and I'm thirty-two years old. This current manic episode has persisted for over a month.

This isn't the first time my odd behaviors have been misunderstood and led me to be treated as a criminal. I know how it works to be booked into custody, and this time was no different; except this time, in my altered state of mind, I couldn't follow or understand the officers' commands. My inability to follow their orders was taken as defiance, and suddenly I was surrounded. Arms bent back, handcuffs squeezing my wrists, voices yelling, the weight of multiple men on my back. The guards escorted me to a secure location.

So here I am, in solitary confinement. I am in dire need of psychiatric intervention. I'm having religious delusions, and in my mind, the world is coming to an end. I have lost my grasp on reality. I am covered in my own urine and feces.

But rather than get me the help I so desperately need, the guards are instead standing outside in the hallway, laughing and joking about my mental state.

"What a nut!" one guard says. "Damn, he is pissing all over himself."

The others start laughing and yell into the safe cell, tapping on the only window. "Crazy... Wacko... Lunatic..." they're taunting. I hear someone else say "nine-one-eight" in a deep, gruff voice.

I yell for help often, however, I don't think they understand the sounds muttering from my dry, cracked lips. There is a metallic taste in my mouth worsening by the second. I try to raise my arm to signal distress, but my arm doesn't respond. Just one drop of water, I pray.

I'm in a dream state, elevated euphoria and the sharpest awareness I've experienced in my life. This must be heaven. I'm caught between two worlds. One world is magnificent, and I am a champion and fearless; in the other, I am frightened and damaged. The longer I am caged, the worse my mania gets.

I lay here, motionless on the floor, my limbs twisted in a bizarre posture. I don't know how long I've been here, but this out-of-body experience has left me exhausted. Suddenly, my breathing is shallow. I get a tingly feeling in my arm, and the cement walls start closing in on me. My vision is spotty.

I am alone.

I hear a whisper, "Are you okay?" I don't know who it is, but the female voice reassures me that everything will be okay. I try to open my eyes and speak, but I can't. It's like someone has shut off the lights. Darkness falls. I hear the voice again, "Get an ambulance! Now!" I feel a cold splash of liquid on my stiff body. I am hauled out of the safe cell, put on a stretcher and boosted into an ambulance. They race me to the nearest hospital.

A great celestial battle is being waged for my soul. The forces of darkness oppose the forces of light. I am broken and wounded, strapped to a hospital bed, isolated from everything I know. My crumbs of hope are the Bible and my faith. God is the source of all light. I recall The Good Book as having many people communicating in the spiritual realm. My repetitive thoughts are of the New and Old Testaments. Noah, Moses, Elijah, Daniel, and even Jesus heard voices. God is communicating with me.

Now I'm labeled seriously mentally ill (SMI). The statistics say more than 10 million Americans have bipolar disorder. During episodes, some people experience hallucinations or delusions. My psychotic symptoms tend to reflect my extreme mood. I have a grand feeling that I am called by the Lord to bear witness to those surrounding me.

At the hospital, the fluorescent lights flicker as I drift in and out of consciousness. Sluggishly, my eyes stretch to open. My vision is a murky haze. I squint and count, 1… 2… 3… Then a dim shadow falls, and it's dark again. I don't know how long my body has been restrained to the bed or how long a watchman has been at my side on high alert, but now I lie pale and lifeless. I am delirious and in kidney failure due to the limited fluid in my body.

In my mind, a glow from my boyhood comes into focus. I am singing in a small country church, wearing my Sunday best. My tiny hands encompass the microphone like a superstar.

Flip… I'm holding my first guitar, placing my hand on the neck, feeling the fretboard with my fingers. My heart dances like a peacock on a rainy day. I can relate to the music when I can't relate to anyone else.

Flip… I'm on stage for the first time, playing the banjo. The audience applause hits an ear-piercing crescendo on the final song. I'm a natural on stage, everyone says.

Flip, flip… I'm at the church for my parent's fortieth wedding anniversary. They're having a ceremony to renew their vows, and the whole family is dressed up. My sisters sit on a pew in the front. I see my nieces and nephews all in a row.

Then, a spine-chilling black shadow pulls down the curtain, bringing my thoughts to a deep, dark, claustrophobic close.

An estimated 50 million people nationwide suffer from some kind of mental disorder. Statistics show one in five Americans struggle with some kind of mental health issues. The best news is that 90% of them are treatable.

Today is the time to begin and continue your healing, to learn new ways of looking deep within the layers of yourself. Say yes to the impulse to grow, expand and embrace. You don't have to know how to handle the journey, just be open to a new understanding.

In the book *A Beautiful Mind*, Sylvia Nasar wrote a classic biography about the mystery of the human mind's triumph over adversity and the healing power of love. The book is about John Nash and his paranoid schizophrenia. He endures delusional episodes, shock therapy and antipsychotic medication. The book was made into a movie and directed by Ron Howard.

John Nash once said, "The only thing greater than the power of the mind is the courage of the heart."

# Family Ties

March 14, 2012, 6:13 A. M. CST

The phone rings at my bedside, drawing me out of my peaceful slumber. Drowsy, I reach for the phone.

"Hey, sis, you called me?"

I'm suddenly wide awake, my frustration immediately rising. "Peter!" I choke out. "Hell yeah, I called! Where have you been? Everyone is scared to death something happened to you! What the HELL is going on?"

My younger brother tells his story at such hyper speed that he has to repeat it several times before I understand. "As I said, I was in a parking lot when a security guard told me to leave. I refused, because I had the right to be there and I was staying.

"The sheriff department came out and arrested me, and they towed my car. They booked me for trespassing, but then released me hours later. I was thirty miles from home, with no car! They finally agreed to give me a ride home after I laid on the ground in front of the police station and refused to move. I've been up all night."

Terror grips my body. *This can't be happening again.* I try to keep my voice steady. "Are you okay? Where are you now?" I ask.

"Sure, sis, I'm fine. I'm exhausted, but I'm fine. I'm back here at the apartment."

"Are you sure you are in a safe place?" I ask, concerned. "I'm very worried about you."

"Yes, I am safe," he says. "I'm just tired. I'm really sorry I woke you up so early. I know you have to work in few hours."

"Listen to me carefully, Peter. You need to get some sleep. It's been a long night. Lock your door and take some Tylenol PM. Call me when you wake up, okay? Promise?"

My request is met with silence.

"Peter, please," I beg. "Promise you will call me when you wake up."

After a suspicious pause, Peter says, "Sure, of course I'll call you, sis. I promise."

Before I can respond, Peter has hung up. I am unaware, but this is the last time I or any of my family members will talk to Peter for weeks to come.

As I'm trying to absorb what just happened, I tap out my parents' number on my phone. After a few rings, my father's deep, drowsy voice answers, "Hello?"

"Hi Dad, it's Cindy. I'm really sorry to call so early."

"That's okay," He yawns. "What is it?"

"I just heard from Peter."

"Peter?" I can hear the fear rise in his voice with just that one word.

"Dad, he was arrested last night for trespassing, and his car has been impounded. He says he's okay, though, and that he's at his apartment now."

He takes a deep breath and exhales slowly. I can hear my mother, Kathryn, beside my dad pleading, "What about Peter? Please, what is she saying?"

"Just a minute, Kathryn," he says to her. "Are you sure he's at the apartment? Wait… I'm putting your mom on the phone."

After a short pause, I hear her raw voice, desperate for information. "Cindy, what is it? What's happened to Peter?"

"He called me just a few minutes ago," I tell her. I recount the story for her. "He promised he would rest, but he was talking so fast. He sounded delusional, Mom."

"He's manic again," she says, fear in her voice. She knows in her heart that it's true.

"Yes, I believe he is. Mom, I think you and Dad should pack up and get to Arizona–"

"We'll leave in an hour," she interrupts. Her voice is breaking, and I hear her choke back a sob. "He has to be okay, Cindy," she bemoans. "He just has to!"

As I hang up I think, *I'm not so sure this time, Mom.*

It is a fourteen-hour trip to Arizona from Oklahoma. I think about my parents and what they're doing right now: making a list of things they might need for the ride, hurriedly packing their bags, certainly forgetting a toothbrush, or maybe socks or shampoo. I imagine the pain of those steps to the car, and my dad behind the wheel, bellowing a prayer to God for his only living son's safety.

I call my sister to fill her in, and the whole family is now on high alert.

This has obviously happened before, more than once. We should have talked about an emergency plan before. But of course we didn't, because we are the typical dysfunctional American family. So here we are, in the middle of an emergency, having to figure out the best way to help Peter from 1000 miles away.

Our family isn't really known for its effective communication or for trusting one another. Approaching each other openly, honestly and respectfully just isn't part of our family dynamic. But what we as a team do have going for us are our opinions. And *oh*, do we have our opinions. We all have different viewpoints, values, ideas and experiences. As I stress to my parents and sister, our diversity can either be disastrous, or it can be a blessing. Let's use it to come up with a cooperative plan, and work together diplomatically to meet our common goal—to help Peter.

This time has come for Someone to take the lead on our mission. I dig my heels in and begin family treatment the hard way. My instinct is to use what I know.

So, I draw up a plan with the seven rules of for working through a problem:

1. Recognize the problem.

2. Examine and expand all the details.

3. Identify alternatives for resolving or managing the problem.

4. Decide on the best solution and implement it.

5. Evaluate the plan.

6. Educate yourself and others about the problem, the solution, and how to handle it next time.

7. Determine your overall success and feel accomplished of your problem-solving.

As I speak to my parents on their way to Arizona, we fall into old patterns, my mother talking at me instead of to me. With every word, my mind fills with these thoughts:

*Inhale. Exhale.*

*Don't let yourself get tangled up in past drama.*

*Inhale. Exhale.*

*Why does Mom criticize all the time?*

*Trust someone.*

*Why do we run amok?*

*Focus on the here and now.*

The resistance walls began to fracture in every corner. The secrets, stigma and dark demons are the foundation of this structure. The quick fixes of medication no longer work. The horizontal cracks in the foundation are a sign of a heavy load. The crooked doorways of confusion, unbalanced manic episodes; it is time to seek professional help.

Silence can be, and often is, deadly.

Our crisis begins on red alert. *Step one, identify the problem. Peter is manic again and needs help.*

I make notes to guide each negotiation on the phone. *Step two, gather information. I make sure to mention Peter's diagnosis, his home address, his last known location, etc.*

After several calls back and forth to various authorities, we know all of our options. *Step three, identify ways to solve the problem.*

Our closets are full of skeletons. Domestic violence. Addiction. Sexual abuse. Mental illness. Infidelity. Sexual orientation. Peter's battle with bipolar disorder seems to be a curse of our DNA. My sister and I are worried. How are our elderly parents going to survive this situation?

Mom and Dad were both born into poverty in 1940s rural Oklahoma; my mother was the seventh of eight children, and my dad was the youngest of two. I recall stories of Mom being bullied because of her clothing, her last name and the kind of food she brought in her lunch pail. My dad tells childhood stories of his self-destructive behavior: truancy, running away from home, drinking and finally dropping out of school. His father signed paperwork for Dad to join the National Guard in 1954, at the ripe old age of fourteen. His hope was to help his youngest find discipline in his life. But after Dad was discharged, the self-destructive patterns continued.

My dad started drinking alcohol at a very young age to cope with the chaos that surrounded him. He married my mother in 1963; she was sixteen, he twenty-three. Sometimes I still look through our old family photos. My dad is younger than I ever remember him being, but he has the slim build I remember, with his arms covered in tattoos from his army days. He always smelled of Old Spice and cigarettes, and his hair was so unruly that it needed a dab of VO5 every day. My mom was lanky with long legs and a slim frame. She is a natural beauty. In her younger years, she felt awkward because she was the tallest girl in the class, but in her wedding photos, her height served her well.

They raised us four children—Cheryl, Cindy, Bobby, Peter— on a modest salary. Although my father quit drinking when I was little, he and my mom were both physically and emotionally abusive to us. It was tearing our family apart, but we kept our pain hidden from those outside the family. Over time, I knew I could no longer allow things with my family to go on as they were. I could no longer allow myself to be abused. I didn't see my parents for many years, but more on that later. I shut them out of my life as I tried to save myself, to work on forging better, healthier relationships in my life.

Everything changed when my brother Bobby died in 2000 from a car accident. I realized that alienating my parents wasn't helping me heal. I had lost Bobby; I didn't want to risk losing the rest of my family forever. The only thing that would truly lead to my healing would be to try to repair the damaged relationship with my parents. When I finally contacted them and shared with them my wish for healing, they were finally more accepting of a safer, more comfortable atmosphere and open conversations about the past. But it had taken years to bridge the gap. Faith, patience and hope helped us heal and grow as a family. God does indeed exist, and this was the proof.

We had saved our family. Now we needed to save Peter.

My parents, my sister and I all have our individual talents, and we are using them to make and implement our plan. We share our medical histories; we apply our computer expertise, our research capabilities, patience, creativity and prayer. Anything we have to give that could help Peter, we give. There is no time for negative thinking, no time for sadness.

As my parents drive, the first thing my sister and I do is write a letter with a description of Peter and his condition, as well as our contact information. We tackle the huge task of faxing and emailing it to police departments, district attorneys' offices and anyone else who might come into contact with him. It is our duty to warn them of Peter's condition for the safety of himself and others in his path. We try to get someone, anyone, to listen. We try to file a missing person report but are unsuccessful. All we want to do is find our brother and get him the help he needs, but no one will help us. We are awakened to the harsh reality of the stigma of mental illness. *We have to keep moving forward. Step four.*

The police department is cold and uncooperative. They are more interested in arresting criminals than helping their citizens or preventing a crisis. The research we find on law enforcement and the dismissive way they handle the mentally ill is disturbing. However, apparently a handful of officers do have crisis intervention training (CIT). They teach that crisis intervention is about people, about our community, our families, our friends and our loved ones. CIT is founded on beliefs that all deserve dignity, understanding, kindness, hope and dedication. We can only hope that one of these trained officers will find our loved one.

Three days later the police call. Peter has been found. He had gone out the wrong exit door of a bank, gotten into a bank employee's car and started scuffling papers around, prompting a clerk to call the police. A sense of relief washes over me, and in my most diplomatic sister voice I plead with the officer to get an evaluation on him as quickly as possible because of his mental state. I speak to him about my brother's erratic, out-of-control hypomania and inflated, grandiose visions. I tell him I'm afraid he will lose his grip with reality and hurt himself or someone else if he doesn't get a medical intervention. I desperately plead for a rescue, ending the conversation by alerting them that my parents are traveling from Oklahoma.

He assures me that Peter will be evaluated and that he will call me back with the results. After we hang up, I wait in panic as the clock ticks unending inside my head. *Step four continues.*

I'm relieved to know he is safe and soon an intervention will take place. I phone the family and inform them as to his status.

It seems that all of our prayers have been answered. Peter will be safe and get the inpatient services he needs.

But my relief is short-lived.

The officer calls me back and tells me that the fire department has examined him, and they determined that Peter showed no signs of erratic behavior and there was no reason to believe he would harm himself or others. They told Peter of our worry, and that he should contact us immediately. Then they let him go.

They let him go.

As of now, Peter hasn't contacted us. I bet he has lost his phone.

I'm stunned that the police had the fire department, which is untrained in dealing with and recognizing mental illness, evaluate my brother. I'm even more stunned that they would let him go before ever even contacting us, knowing that we are desperate to find him, and that my parents drove all the way from Oklahoma to find him. I have hung up with the police officer, and I don't even remember what I've said to him. I wasn't gentle, though; I do know that. This was our chance to find Peter, and to get him the intervention he so desperately needs, and now he's gone again. It is incomprehensible. The police seem to have just gone through the motions to placate me, to get rid of me.

This is the cold, hard truth about how people with mental illness are treated in this country. Having a neurotransmitter disorder such as bipolar, a disturbance in your brain, the struggle can be terrifying. And it is met with incompetency.

I try to dissect the information forwards and backwards. My thoughts become foggy, muddled.

Hurt.

Everyone hurts, but our family has had an abundance of it.

One generation after another, this secret, relentless grief has been unearthed. But going through it has been a type of baptism. Each negative experience has awoken a yearning for peace, love and change. This yearning now guides my path.

But this distress, this endeavor of trying to find and help Peter, triggers my own past struggles. I had worked hard to overcome my negative self-esteem, thinking I wasn't good enough. It's hard to give up old habits, to give up the old family rules of "don't talk" and "don't feel." I realize that not only am I grieving for Peter, I am also grieving my own childhood. But I remind myself, that is the past. The pursuit of peace and progress is what carries me forward.

One of my favorite sayings is by Eleanor Roosevelt. "It isn't enough to talk about peace. One must believe in it. And it isn't enough to believe in it. One must work at it."

How do you find peace in a situation like this?

Never give up. You are not alone, I say to myself over and over, hour after hour, day after day.

I have to take a break from this sadness. So I put everything down and walk out the door, down the street to a park. I sit under a big elm tree, the shade giving me relief and the sun giving me warmth. I'm feeling a deep sadness in my core being.

I meditate as I was taught many years ago. I fall into a self-guided tour to a happier place.

My earliest childhood memory of internal happiness is playing in our homemade tree house outside my childhood home. The trunk held up the branches as it pushed toward the sunlight. The tree of happiness again makes its way into my conscience.

The roots of the tree anchor it to the earth, keeping it stable. They draw nutrients and chemicals from the soil and use them to grow, develop and restore.

They are strength. They are survival.

I reflect on the long personal journey I have made, out of the chaos and into peace. I realize that one of the only constants in life is change. Just as the weather has different seasons, our lives have different seasons; we have joy, sorrow, hardship and preparation.

After meditating, I walk back to my house and reenter the chaos and a different reality.

I turn on my computer to listen to the online radio. I grab my journal and pen, sit in my office chair and try to think as Peter might. I start writing: *If I needed help, where would I go? How would I live without money? Where would I go for shelter? How would I change my clothes? Where would I shower?*

Suddenly, from the radio comes the song "Where No One Stands Alone" by Allison Krauss. The lyrics fill my soul.

> *Hold my hand all the way,*
> *Every hour, every day,*
> *From here to the great unknown.*
> *Take my hand; let me stand*
> *Where no one stands alone.*

I know facing life can be hard at times and facing it alone is much harder. My brother is alone. Alone and sick.

The phone rings. It is my parents calling to inform me that they are nearing the Arizona border.

What is happening to us is a family's worst nightmare. This must happen to hundreds, maybe thousands of us across the United

States every month. A person cries out daily in crisis. This is not just our family's story. It is a story told across all barriers and borders.

Mental illness can strike anyone. It knows no age limit, economic status, race, creed or color. Bipolar disorder is characterized by debilitating mood swings. It affects approximately 12.6 million individuals in the United States, according to the World Health Organization's Global Burden of Disease study of 2004.

♦♦♦♦

**Journaling Questions:**

1.  Why am I afraid of change?

    _____
    _____
    _____
    _____
    _____
    _____
    _____
    _____

2.  Why am I afraid of failure?

    _____
    _____
    _____
    _____
    _____
    _____
    _____
    _____

3.  Do I deserve a happy, healthy lifestyle?

    _____
    _____
    _____
    _____
    _____
    _____
    _____
    _____

4. Why do people make changes in their lives?

_____
_____
_____
_____
_____
_____
_____
_____

5. What does my tree of happiness look like?

_____
_____
_____
_____
_____
_____
_____
_____

6. Why am I afraid of success?

_____
_____
_____
_____
_____
_____
_____
_____

7. Do I need help?

_____
_____
_____
_____
_____
_____
_____
_____

8. When I look in a mirror, what do I see?

_____
_____
_____
_____
_____
_____
_____
_____
_____
_____
_____

9. How can I make a crisis plan?

_____
_____
_____
_____
_____
_____
_____
_____
_____
_____

10. Is there CIT training in my city?

_____
_____
_____
_____
_____
_____
_____
_____
_____
_____

# The Journey

March 16, 2012, 4:30 P.M. CST

My parents finally arrive at Peter's apartment in Arizona. They go to management and ask them to open the apartment for a welfare check.

On the phone later, they tell me that Peter's place is a wreck. It is clear that he believes the world is ending. *Hypomania.*

Every drain is plugged, and a hose runs out of the kitchen faucet. Every room is a disaster. There is cereal poured on the shower floor. Big piles of clothing are everywhere, and it looks like more than one person might be staying there. Several treasured stringed instruments are left on the floor with neglect, while trivial, common items like notebooks, shoes, and food are displayed prominently.

My parents find pieces of paper everywhere filled with his writing. Most of the words aren't legible, but those that are show a man with religious delusions of grandeur and a heightened sense of self-worth. He writes that he's had special messages from God and has been elected by God to save humanity. He believes that he is John the Baptist and that "All life will end on Earth. Destruction is coming, and no one is safe."

There is no way for my parents to deny his diagnosis, with this bizarre dysfunction staring them right in the face.

Their world has been turned upside-down. Things are worse than we had expected.

Peter is indeed missing.

They sit on the sofa and weep together.

When the tears have run dry, they kneel and pray for divine intervention. Medicine, hospitalization, faith and love can save their only living son from himself.

If loving someone to wellness were possible, Peter would be healed. He is a charming, gentle, brilliant man, envied for his talents and stage presence. Living a life with bipolar disorder is living a life of contradiction. The brain that makes Peter a danger to himself and others is the same brain that makes him so charismatic and full of life.

But right now, his life must be a living hell.

My parents felt indescribable pain when my brother Bobby died. Peter's disappearance has brought them face-to-face with those past feelings once again, immobilizing them with the fear that they will lose yet another child. I'm afraid that they can't bear living through it again.

At this point, our entire family has questioned their beliefs. Among the four of us, there is the minister, the woman with passion for Christ, the spiritually connected, and the loner. How do we understand God in a situation like this? How can we trust in Him when one of his children is suffering as Peter is? But we've come to realize that we need to trust in God to make our way in this world. It is the only way.

That is very hard to do when you're feeling guilty and overwhelmed. Although Peter has been prescribed medications for his illness, we know he hadn't been taking them faithfully; yet we ignored the signs and continued to enable him. We refuse to face his (and our) reality.

How do we find the positive when confronted with so much negative? It is a question we're all facing during this chaos. Finding clarity in this madness seems impossible.

But there has to be a breaking point. Things are either going to get better, or they are going to get worse. With the signs of stress beginning to show—sleeplessness, anxiety, disorientation and depression—finding the energy to fight gets harder and harder. But the tears have become our motivation. We've hit that breaking point, and we refuse to take no for an answer.

We've rekindled the fire and are tackling our mission with a newfound energy. We are putting in long hours, sometimes as much as sixteen hours a day, doing internet research, talking to professionals, and doing anything we can to find Peter.

*Continue step four.* My parents meet with the Arizona affiliate of the National Alliance on Mental Illness (NAMI) on Tuesday night for guidance and support from people who have experienced and survived the same nightmare. Mental illness, it seems, knows no boundaries.

They have roamed the streets and parks of Arizona in desperation, looking for any signs of Peter. Plenty of transients have their own stories about Peter—he was on drugs, he was with this girl —but everyone's story is different. They can put no stock into what these people are saying.

My father talks to the strange, old, gray-headed man handing out cold meals. The man speaks some words of wisdom about God and his strength, then returns to his mission of feeding the homeless. My parents return to Peter's apartment, depleted and alone, no stone left unturned.

We're again beginning to lose hope. With all of our efforts and desperation, it seems that no help is coming. But we cannot give up. We must fight for Peter. God knows no one else will.

Bipolar is a particular kind of pain, elation, loneliness and terror rolled into one. There is a tremendous high. Power and intensity drive the mania. Then it changes. The ideas are too fast, too many, too confusing.

We all face adversity, and we either persevere or fall short. All our lives we've been taught that it's all in your heart. You just need more willpower and self-control and you can overcome anything. But with bipolar episodes there is no control. My brother Peter has a disease. Willpower can't conquer this disease any more than it can conquer cancer. Too often, people with mental illness are dismissed as "crazy," instead of being seen for what they truly are: terribly ill.

In the coming days, we all weep. My mother, my father, my sister, my nieces and nephews and I all weep out of fear and out of helplessness.

My parents visit with people around the property of Peter's apartment. They contact towing companies to locate his car. I call all of the hospitals, jails and shelters within a fifty-mile radius of Peter's town. I map out a search area, call the crisis hotline, and consider posting flyers on convenience stores and telephone poles. I even think of trying to file another missing person report. Anything we can think of, we do. Now desperate, we see everything as a clue, and we are prepared to follow every one of them to find an indication of where he's gone. It is becoming impossible to see through all of the information we've gathered to see the facts, to see the truth.

We drift in and out of our own guilt. We are vulnerable and alone, just as Peter must be. We are living on the ragged edge of a cliff. Darkness has fallen upon us all once again, swallowing our hope.

It is night, and I'm lying curled up in my bed, crying. The tears give way to exhaustion, and I slowly drift off to sleep.

The dream I have is out-of-the-ordinary for me. I am not a visionary of religious encounters, so this is a first.

A hearty, white chrysanthemum is in full bloom. As I draw closer to the flower, I see that the petals have transformed into a band of angels, hundreds of them. Each angel touches the next with its interlocking wings. It is an optical illusion. I am just a passerby, gazing.

Their androgynous, luminous spirits are powerful soldiers for the good of mankind. They are truly benevolent, celestial beings with extraordinary beauty that generates warm, healing light. The presence of the Divine is within reach. I think of grace, kindness, attainment and harmony.

Looking more closely, I notice that one of the angels looks different. It has no wings. I simply bow my head in reverence.

The angels' draping robes are translucent tapestry. They glisten with each flicker of light, with just a twist of sparkle.

There is an odor of sweet fragrance in the air. Then, encompassed by his comrades, my brother Peter appears, surrounded by love. I am filled with joy as this revelation comes to me: *being alone is impossible in a world full of angels.*

And I'm awake.

This vision is my spiritual awakening.

I've always believed in a higher power other than myself, but have never really believed it was there, waiting for me. I always wanted to believe I was something God made, my heart believed but my mind did not. Now, in this connectedness, it is flowing like a small brook, joining together with larger ones to make a river, a waterway to my soul.

The Divine made Its presence known.

The next morning I replay the dream for my mother. We both know this is a sign. A miracle is coming. Suddenly, we are both at peace.

We both pause in the silence for a moment. I gather my thoughts and burst out excitedly, "Angels don't appear for small stuff. This must be something big! This must be a delivery of true importance."

I am thankful for and inspired by this unique gift, this visit from the Divine.

The morning comes with a sun-soaked sky. A new day unfolds. This is our golden opportunity to complete what we were unable to do yesterday. We inhale, exhale, and enjoy the swell of confidence in our extraordinary efforts.

It has now been five or six days since any of us have heard from Peter. With the help of a local social worker, my parents file for guardianship of their son. *Still step four.* This guardianship is a major step to ensure our sanity. Someone is finally listening, and just maybe, we can find my brother.

It's been a couple of days since the court filed the documents. Yesterday, my parents received a call requesting their presence to meet with the judge assigned to the guardianship case.

They are at the courthouse in an unfamiliar place, 1000 miles away from their home, from their comfort zone. They speak to the judge about guardianship of their thirty-two-year-old son. The judge asks a few personal questions, then approves the document.

Then the news comes. They have located Peter. He is in the hospital, and he is having kidney failure.

My parents are devastated. The lost has been found, and he is near death.

The judge grants my parents permission to go see Peter at the hospital, now that he is their ward. When they arrive at the front desk of the hospital, the nurse picks up the phone and mutters into the receiver, then asks them to wait there. Soon, a police officer appears and informs them that they are not allowing any visitors. His voice is cold and unemotional.

Frustrated, my father insists that the officer call to confirm the guardianship. The officer calls the Chief of Police, but he also denies consent to see Peter. They feel defeated. They have come so far, Peter is there, just steps away from them, and they are being kept from him. I wonder if God has left them to fend for themselves in this moment. They relinquish, knowing they will not win this battle tonight.

How they found the strength to leave without seeing Peter, I can never know. I can't imagine the sorrow they feel with each step they had to take, walking away from him. How do you find the strength to leave your only living son, suffering and lifeless?

This is a trial of their faith. These faith-filled, small town folks have taken God at His word and are facing this tribulation head-on, forging through the wall of fire.

Day in and day out, they read their Bible and pray. They are following their faith and standing firmly with their religious beliefs. Three days have passed, and my parents still haven't been allowed to communicate with Peter. But they are prepared for a long-term walk with God, making slow and steady progress, like the story of the tortoise and the hare. Stick with God and the truth will be revealed.

My parents are suspicious. Why would the police refuse to let relatives with an order of guardianship into Peter's hospital room? My sister and I are dumbfounded when they tell us. They are right to be suspicious.

The next day, my parents speak with Steve, the social worker, and fill him in. He is cautionary about the police department and their handling of mental illness cases. He says he will try to get an intervention team to evaluate Peter's mental and physical needs, but this will take time and lots of effort. Getting someone committed is a complicated procedure. Is it a voluntary or involuntary commitment? Would a person with mental illness understand his or her need for psychiatric treatment?

This has become a crisis beyond our scope. We have to let the professionals handle it from here. They insist that they'll keep us updated daily until Peter is allowed a transfer to a mental hospital for evaluation. *Step five, evaluate the plan. We found Peter and my parents obtained guardianship. The plan was successful but it could have gone better were there fewer obstacles and adversaries.*

The day is finally here. Mom and Dad are going to see Peter today.

They walk into the hospital, seeing their son for the first time since they arrived in Arizona. They are shocked at Peter's appearance. He is barely recognizable. He has lost weight, and he is still erratic. His brain has declared war on his body; he is drooling and unable to communicate with them. His blue eyes are empty and set deep in his head. He looks as though he could be a transient—unshaven face, unruly hair, and ill-fitting clothes. They think he has recognized them as his parents, though, so that gives them hope. The visit is cut short to let Peter rest, but before leaving, Mom and Dad visit with the staff and give them their contact numbers. They go to see Peter daily, and they see regular progress. Although he is communicating better and is mostly lucid, at times he still exists in another realm. He is even able to talk to me on the phone occasionally, and although he is hard to understand much of the time, I am grateful that he is there to talk to. He tells me he sees our dead siblings, which worries me that maybe he is approaching the end of his life. I call frequently to check on his progress with staff members. They have changed his medications so many times that it is hard to keep up with the names and dosages. He has been transported to the hospital more than once, due to drug interactions and overdose.

*Step six, educate yourself and others.* There are certain stigmas about mental illness (MI) in America. How do you talk about it with friends and family members when it is either not taken seriously or seen as a personal weakness?

When a person with MI finally speaks up and shares their experiences, they are often accused of being lazy or weak-minded, and told they just need to "snap out of it" and try harder. Because of this, millions of Americans suffer silently, too embarrassed and afraid to ask for help. Instead, they try to function as though nothing is wrong and fail to get the treatment they so desperately need. MI is a brain disorder—a physical disease, just as diabetes or Parkinson's disease are—and must be treated as such. Just because you can't see the symptoms with your eyes, doesn't mean it's not real. This is why MI is known as an invisible disease. There are no pink or yellow ribbon days for it.

But even though MI affects a person's brain function, which is apparent in their behaviors, the disease does not define the person. To support someone with mental illness, you must see the individual first, not the illness. We can find strength in sharing our experiences with others. When we share, we care. If we can draw from each others' knowledge, we can find solutions.

Because of the stigma surrounding MI, seeking treatment at a mental hospital can seem shameful and embarrassing. But in life, sometimes we need assistance, and this is just one option, one way to figure things out under the care of trained professionals.

People with MI should not be made to feel like failures because of their disease. We need to find our voices and make our towns, states and country recognize that fifty million people in our country struggle daily.

To quote the first sentence of one of my favorite books, The Road Less Traveled by M.Scott Peck. M.D., "Life is difficult."

I have learned that if we expect a life with no pain, no heartache, no death, or no affliction, we will be sorely disappointed.

My family's story is just one of hundreds. If you are reading this book, you probably have your own story of struggles.

There are millions of people raising kids, working and functioning in society who have been diagnosed with mental disorders. Some people are working very hard to break the stigma. It is okay to take an active stand and be counted.

*Step seven, empowerment.* My brother Peter survived this crisis. After several weeks and more trips to the hospital, he was released and my parents brought him back to Oklahoma to be cared for by our family. I am happy to report, during the writing of this book, that he is happy and healthy and he manages his bipolar disorder faithfully. He is well-liked in his community, and our family is so proud of his victories. His life is ordinary for a thirty-seven year old guy. He plays music, and he dates.

He lives in an apartment and takes care of all of his own needs. He is financially responsible. We enjoy good times together. He does not let his mental disorder define him.

It took commitment from all of us at different times. There were many struggles as we all went through stages of grief. My parents' faith grew even stronger. They still grieve and weep and trust and pray because they know the true meaning of miracles.

This does not happen for all families. There are known cases of abuse and even death because of the mishandling of mental disorders. Across the United States, staff working in jails and prisons use unnecessary, excessive, and even malicious force against prisoners with mental health disabilities, said the Human Rights Watch team. The U.S. Justice Department also cites multiple examples of police mishandling a crisis.

"Officers too often use unreasonable force against individuals with mental illness, individuals in a medical crisis and individuals with impaired faculties," according to a 58-page letter of findings addressed to Mayor Frank Jackson in Cleveland, Ohio. U.S. Attorney General Eric Holder and the Justice Department delivered a scathing review of the Cleveland Police Department's use-of-force policies and practices. During a press conference at the U.S. District Court in Cleveland in 2014, Holder insisted that sweeping reforms must be put in place.

We must help to educate everyone about this public health crisis in our country. Public officials need adequate training on crisis intervention.

We should not accept less. If we can't educate the public on mental illness, we fail everyone.

·

# Mental Evaluation

*I need help.* It is my belief those are the three hardest words to say.

My name is Cindy.

Rewind a half a century, and that is where my story begins.

I was the second of four children. My sister, Cheryl, is the oldest, then me. Bobby came along five years later and Peter, who could have been a prodigy, came eight years after that.

Neither of my parents graduated from high school. My mother was sixteen and my dad twenty-three when they got married in 1963. I was born eleven months after my sister. I always felt like I was an accident. I was born into struggle.

I'm on the middle of the introvert scale.

I've always liked solitude.

My mother excused my behavior as "shy" when I was younger. I hated to talk because I had a stutter. I attended speech therapy when I started school to improve my speech impediment.

People told me that I was wise beyond my years. That I was an old soul.

But I wandered aimlessly. I thought mostly about my security. Scared and trusting of no one.

I pretended to be brave for my siblings who leaned on me, but really, I was terrified, too.

My father was alcoholic until I was five. We didn't realize what this meant until much later in life.

I always wanted to fit in. I wanted friends, but I didn't know how to communicate outside of my own head.

My mother once identify me as a "loner."

Sometime around kindergarten, my dad was saved and became a Christian. We started going to church. We learned of God. We went to Sunday School. We sang "Jesus Loves Me."

I had loved nature since a young age.

I spent much of my free time on a tree platform with my brother, Bobby. We were closest.

That tree with Bobby was the first place I can ever remember experiencing internal joy. The trunk held us up high on the branches as we constructed our tranquility. The wooden platform was nailed with hundreds of nails.

I could feel God in this tree. Yes, God as I knew him. Genuine love!

This tree, without purpose or intent, gave me shade and shelter from the chaos in my childhood. The bark was fractured, coarse and grayish brown. The height reached sixty or sixty-five feet.

It was a creation of God's, just like I was. It was a home for birds, squirrels, bugs and me. I would lie, nestled in my home, and feel the sunlight welcoming my spirit. I examined every part of this elm. The green leaves were oval and came to a point at one end. There were lines down the middle of each leaf, and their sides were jagged. I would climb my way to God every time I would lose heart or feel anxious. This was my first realization that there would, eventually, be a time for everything.

I think I was in fourth or fifth grade when my father opened his church. The place of worship was a small congregation in the middle of the bad side of town.

We went to church plenty. We had revivals. We sang old hymns. We studied the Bible.

I was a preacher's kid.

Later, I was in a prison of a different kind, trapped in the pain of chronic depression with no way out.

I remember a sermon about there being a time for birth, a time to die; a time to plant and a time to harvest. This lodged itself in my conscience. It became a lens through which I could understand the world around me.

I would think of all the things God made while I was sitting in my nest, created of boards and nails. The jagged green leaves intrigued me. They whispered to me, or so I pretended. The steady breeze gave them a language only I could understand. Each fall, the leaves would turn yellowish and plummet to the ground. Then the old elm tree looked barren. But after the hardship winter, the tree and its leaves emerged again for the spring season. After the flowering, there were always plenty of elm seeds. And the umbrella tree of shade returned.

I remember talking about trees in my grade school class.

I decided that trees would be my favorite thing. One of my teachers said "a tree is living, dying and dead, all at the same time."

This is where the tree of happiness was born.

◆◆◆◆

It's later, and I'm twenty-five years old. I'm in a mental hospital, here for a psychological evaluation. I am physically restrained, and my mind is still in an altered, gray state. The scent of ammonia consumes the hallways.

This is when I noticed that I had crossed over, into a new understanding. My thinking has changed, my voice seems different and I have no emotion. I am a disconnected, jumbled mess. No one understands what I am saying. The communication between one world and the other is impossible.

The warm sensation of pee runs down my leg as I sit, shivering, in the small intake room. An undersized room, eight-by-ten feet, with small desk and a couple of chairs cuts me off from the world. The lonely bookshelf stacked high with hardbacks is clearly the only source of information in this space. There is a metallic and dented, four-drawer file cabinet squeezed into one corner. The lock on the cabinet tells me it must contain confidential patient files.

On the other side of the desk sits a frumpy, middle-aged white woman. Her hair in a bun, long strands of gray hair fall by each ear. Her stooped body language gives me every reason to believe that she doesn't care. She doesn't care about me. She doesn't care about her job. She's just executing the routine.

She shuffles papers and is looking in the desk drawers for a writing utensil when she asks me the first question. She says simply, "Why are you here?"

I am sitting here with piss all over me, and this bitch asks me what I'm doing here?!

Really?!

I am here for an evaluation.

Psychologists use tests and other assessments to measure and observe behavior. But most of the time, when an individual finally gets an evaluation, they are already mentally unstable.

My internal consciousness tries over and over to communicate. The food is scanty, and the fresh water is definitely not fresh.

My mind is a sabotaged cylinder, but my spirit is an iridescent, prophetic, fiery, perfect image of crazy. Behind God and beneath the demons of my destructive self lies an egocentric, cruel, insensitive, deceitful, angry and isolated female.

I am a failure as a young woman.

At the center of my core is a secret. If people knew the truth, they would hate me almost as much as I hate myself. I deserve this mayhem. I deserve to be alone and humiliated, like a solitary badger. My thoughts race so fast that I need forewarning of what will come next, thousands of negative words jumble in no sagacious manner.

I hate myself, and I want to be dead. Lifeless.

Rage. My mind is flooded with thoughts of pure evil. I hate my life. Frenzy. My hands are trembling, and my knees bobble up and down so fast that I can not count the iterations.

I told my therapist, "I need help," that morning in her office. I am wretched with fear because of my daily torture ritual. I am dangerous. I am obsessed. I am a failure full of fear.

The hospital makes me strip down to my underwear and bra. They search my clothes and take out my shoe strings. They look inside my mouth and run their fingers through my hair. It reminds me of television shows were jailhouse officers inspect and frisk their arrestees.

The nurse tells me I can see the doctor in the morning for my evaluation. *Why, do I need an evaluation to kill myself?* I think. She gives me a gown has me dress in front of her. Then whispers my room number and sends me wandering down the hall. The room is small but clean. It looks like a hospital room. I have lost weight and my body seems disfigured in the mirror. I pace aimlessly up and down the corridor, to and from my room. I see lots of other doors on my path down the corridor.

No emotion, no pain. My mind is obsessed with finding something to relieve my internal pain. I look for light bulbs, loose metal, springs from under the bed. My search is bleak. Nothing.

Until I remember I always have a plan B, a secret stash for pain. A safety pin I kept hidden in my bra.

Self harm is a release for people like me.

I take my blanket and pillows from the bed and perch in the closet for a protected space. I start cutting and piercing myself. The blood runs sluggishly down my arm. The white sheet starts to saturate with the red color.

I float off to sleep.

Then, I wake up covered in dried blood. A nurse was standing over me as I lay tangled in a fetal position in the closet.

She asks me for the tool.

I shake my head.

She states they will rip the room apart and call the doctor for a sedative if I do not comply. I give her the cutting device. She helps clean me up and gives me a new gown. She hands me a small medication cup and watches me swallow. I don't know what medication I am given, nor the dosage.

They direct me towards the lounge area where "Group" is being held. I get a cup of water and take my place in the nearest corner. To me this is "hog wash" a bunch of psychos talking about their nutty behavior.

I start losing focus fast. The room starts spinning. Darkness falls upon me.

I wake up in my room with a wet cloth on my head. A nurse's aid is watching over me. I try to sit up but the room gets dizzy again and I notice the drool running down my chin. I try to talk but my words are slurred and tongue feels huge. I am unable to coordinate my movements.

These are the side effects of antipsychotics, I am told. They give me another medication to reduce the side effects. They tell me it will take time to wear off. After a few days of sleeping, I am able to gain control of my movements and walk to the lounge.

There are several other loud, hyper and just plan annoying patients.

There is a classic bitch who really does not give a fuck about anything. Her name is Kara. She weighs about two hundred fifty pounds and keeps to herself. Kara walks around with her fist clenched and often checks the clock. Once, one of the patients got in her way at dinner time, and she punched him in the mouth. He ran off, and she starting kicking as hard as she could at the main doors. She yelled, "Let me out of this fucking hell hole, right... fucking... now!" She is a handful for the mental health workers. She later transfers to another facility.

Then there is Ronald. He sleeps all day and is awake at night. His room smells of ass.

His clothes stink. He is not well-groomed. He hunches his shoulders and looks at the floor most of the time. He has slim build about 6'1". If I guess, he is about thirty. He wears flannel shirts and the fringe on his jeans is tattered. Someone on the floor yells, "Take a fucking shower, you pissed on yourself again!"

There is a pay phone so people can call and talk to patients.

One time a guy named Albert stood at the phone for thirty minutes having a conversation. No one was on the other end.

Albert is a man of medium build with a mustache and a beard. He wears long sleeved shirts that are tailored. His hair is cut short and his facial hair is well-groomed. He wears cologne that I smell every time he passes me in the hallway. Albert has intelligent conversation about social issues and news related topics. He has a slight, closed lip smile and shifty eye contact. He often squeaks this high-pitch laughter. This guy does not shuffle his feet like Ronald.

Carol is a woman dressed in a skirt and nice pressed blouse. She uses make up, lipstick, and eyeliner. She wears expensive shoes and carries a designer purse with her everywhere she goes. She is beautiful, with wavy brown hair, and slim, about a hundred twenty five pounds. She fidgets, sweats, and bites her bottom lip constantly. Her demeanor changes suddenly without warning. She often angrily runs her hands through her hair.

There is lots of yelling and loud noises. One after another, we act out, almost like we know whose turn it is next.

There is one guy... I can't recall his name. He is putting voodoo curses on the staff because he can't get a snack when he wants it. He walks around all day pacing. He shouts "Sonofabitch!" every time he gets to the end of the hallway and has to turn around. He tries to hang around the nurse's station. They are not too impressed with his flirtations behavior. This man has long blinks and unwarranted smiles. He walks around with his hands clasped together over his crotch. A couple of times he was combative, and I saw the veins throbbing in his neck as they came running with an injection. He struggles until the medication kicks in. Yelling... screaming... He is hauled into a special room.

Then, of course, there was an ordinary paranoid schizophrenic on the ward.

He thinks everyone is trying to kill him. His has a muscular build and is about 6'3". This male wrings his hands frequently. He checks food and water all the time. He never walks in front of the window, and he is on hyper alert at all times. He talks to different people all the time, and he often thinks he is invisible. One day I am in the same room, watching him. He is staring into space, rocking back and forth, seated on the sofa.

Ronald spoke to him and says something about the CIA. He twists off! He throws the chairs and knocks over the table. We high-tail it to our rooms, the schizo gets hit with a Haldol shot, and he is under control within minutes.

These are only few of my ward-mates that I recall.

Then there is me. I am shy and constantly peeing on myself. The side effects of the medication were tremors, dry mouth, drooling, pounding heartbeat, anxiety… and confusion. I bury my face in my hands a lot. My droopy body drags my feet along. I keep my distance from others in the group. Then, after a few days when the medication did not work, they start me on a new medication. The cycle of new side effects introduce themselves again. Most of the time, tremors and drooling are always present.

I am of a medium build, about two hundred pounds. I stand 5'9". My clothes are baggy. I do not wear make-up, and my face is pale. I am a simple person. I sob regularly. I often stare wide-eyed at the drama unfolding around me. Obsessively, I tap my fingers over and over again, a subtle gesture of my hyper alertness. I spot the exit every time I walk into a room and form an escape plan in my head.

This is perfect staging for my fight/flight/freeze response.

Several people come to talk to me during this time. I do not recall who they are or why they are talking to me. They ask me questions like, "Who is the president of the United States?" I say, "Well, Clinton, if I remember right." They use their pens to mark something on a paper.

Then other questions:

"Have you been sick?"

"Have you recently hit your head?"

"Do you drink alcohol or do drugs?"

They put another mark on the paper.

They ask me what brought me to this facility.

I do not answer most of their questions.

I can only catch one or two words, then get distracted and lose my concentration.

It is like I am being interrogated again and again.

I yell, "I JUST WANT TO DIE!!! If you can't help me, then leave me alone!"

I am constantly looking for loose light bulbs, scrap objects, or cleaner I can ingest. I am on the hunt. Obsessed.

Once I pull the fire alarm. I figure that the janitor will leave the cleaning cart, so I can ingest bleach.

I grab the jug as the siren wails and start to drink it. The staff catches me. This is when I receive my first injection and became 1:1 maximum security. I want to die. The medication puts a damper on my plan.

I am not sure how many days or even weeks I am in this mental health center.

The days grew into more days. In my disorganized thoughts I know I am being treated for a mental illness. There is no physical pain.

My pain is inside.

I want to die.

It is trauma that I carry deep down, inside the core of my being.

I had received a silent message from my parents not to talk about these kinds of things as a child.

I pretend I don't give a damn. This is not a vacation, and there is no happy place here.

I have three words for you right now: *I am wrong.*

So here I am, attached to this burdensome duffel bag of misery. I can't consent to it being unlocked. It is too painful and shameful for anyone to believe. There is only one key, yet I do not posses it.

It is hidden like gold coins beneath the deep dark ocean.

It seems like I am going right while everyone else is going left. I'm here and everyone else is there. I'm surrounded by people I don't know. At this point, I do not have any idea if anyone knows where I am.

I don't remember how I get to the hospital or who brings me here.

My sister visits.

We share our secrets and cry.

I start to miss my kids, but not my husband. I'm not sure I want to return to him.

The medication begins to work. My desire to harm begins to subside. I am released with an appointment with my therapist.

Not a treatment plan. No tools to deal with a crisis. Just an appointment. This used to be the norm. But if you are being treated for a psychiatric condition, how are you supposed to return to normal life without a plan? There needs to be steps. There needs to be goals. There needs to be resources and safeguards.

Many people are uncomfortable with the idea that mental illness is a disease.

Many families don't know where to turn. Their loved ones are sick, and they don't know what to do. No matter how much the family wants the individual to recover, it is not enough. The journey is up to the one with mental illness.

It can't be cured, but it can be managed.

If I had not said those three simple words, "I need help," I may not be alive today.

Every family must know that unless you are part of the solution, you will continue to be part of the problem.

Suffering is difficult.

Many people feel alone and desperate.

Each year, more than 41 thousand individuals take their own lives, leaving behind thousands more friends and family members to navigate the tragedy of their loss.

According to the Alcohol, Drug Abuse, and Mental Health Administration a report from the Secretary Task Force on Youth Suicide, Volume 1: Overview and Recommendation in 1989 publication, suicide is the 10th leading cause of death among adults in the U.S. and the 3rd leading cause of death among fifteen to twenty-four year olds. The U.S. Department of Health & Human Services provides statistics each year.

Suicidal thoughts or behaviors are both damaging and dangerous, and are therefore considered a psychiatric emergency.

# Surviving the Three D's: Divorce

It wasn't a sudden revelation that I had to leave my husband. It wasn't about my sexuality. It wasn't about my children. It was for my own mental health.

For years, I had been living as a young mother in a rural, isolate area, with only him, my children, and my own inner demons.

I was getting better, going to therapy, but in order to continue, I couldn't be around him anymore.

It was horrible. The worst were the court battles for custody of our children. Others believed I was an unsuitable mother because of my mental health struggles, and I tended to agree with them. I used to disappear for days on end when I couldn't take it any more. He was unsuited because he often left them alone. Neither of us could trust the other. Finally, I was given my children back, except my oldest son who chose to live with his father for a time.

While we were together, my husband was controlling and manipulative. In the throws of my illness, I needed someone to be controlling, someone to be in charge.

But not anymore.

Finally leaving and putting money down on my own place was empowering. I finally knew that I wouldn't be back. I could be my authentic self and heal.

I also learned to ask for help. My sister and I had supported each other from a young age, not because we had a lot in common, but because we had to. She was there for me again now.

Slowly, I started to rebuild my life. A new foundation, brick by brick. There were new opportunities, new resources, new inspiration.

Most importantly, I chose to surround myself with people who valued and invested in me. This meant cutting out some friends, even family members.

For about five years, this even meant cutting out my parents.

My decisions were my own.

This time in my life was empowering, inspirational, and absolutely necessary. It was also difficult, chaotic, and exhausting.

My friend, Linda, always told me never to be content with someone else's definition of myself. Instead, she urged me to define *me*. We talked and talked about our quest in life's big adventure. Both of our paths were bumpy at times. But we cheered each other when we followed our own desires towards the place of peace and authenticity that we both knew existed.

We became closer and closer, year after year.

We stayed in touch over thousands of miles of distance with letters and cards. We survived twenty-one years of friendship. We both like written text. We don't often email or talk on the phone. Our friendship has merit because we've been friends in sunshine and in shade.

She read one of the first drafts of this book. I value her opinion.

She dreams of paddling across the state of Michigan. I dream of writing my first novel. Her need for nature and the outdoors—opposite of my need for solitude and pondering philosophical questions—made way for a great friendship. She invested in me as a unique individual. We both started our journeys of self-discovery.

I began to think I could be a mover and a shaker in this world. So I challenged myself to be more involved, more present with this vision. I had to trust the message of happiness that had been presented to me.

I was building a great foundation for my future. Through this experience, I found my voice.

All my life I had been coached to be something different than what I am, had never taken control of my own destiny.

I was now a single mom with four children to support. I had to develop a system to maintain my own mental health.

There were days when I wanted my crazy, distorted life back. But then I would give Linda a call, and she would remind me of the real chaos I had faced in years past.

For once, I could be in control of my own well-being.

I campaigned for honesty and truth. I often gave thanks for my journey. Many people supported me. My family and friends helped guide my transition. They gave me confidence to continue this path so I could be accountable for my own life.

My sister was especially important. She could sometimes be a neutral party. She took my children to see their grandparents when I wouldn't or couldn't.

I think she dissociated from our troubled childhoods. She was only eleven months older, but when we played as kids, she was the teacher and I was the student.

She's on her fourth marriage now, repeating her own difficult cycles. But her career as a nurse means she has always helped others. She is well loved by her patients and staff. We both took our own journeys of struggle and growth. She has always supported me and my transformation.

16 million adults in the United States have a major depressive disorder. Depression can contribute to divorce, and vice versa.

Often with mental illness, one partner withdraws and can no longer support the other. It's also energy-consuming, which doesn't leave much time for the marriage. The stress of mental illness, doctor visits, health insurance coverage, etc., also strain a marriage.

Even antidepressants and other medications can affect a couple's relationship. One common side effect is a lowered libido and/or the inability to orgasm. This is especially prevalent in women and can lead to a dissatisfying, undesirable sex life for both partners.

Dissatisfaction and lack of support in any aspect of a marriage may also lead to infidelity. Infidelity is sometimes the impetus for divorce and has many other negative impacts on a partner's life. In addition, mistrust is a large killer of relationships.

And mental illness isn't just a problem for heterosexual couples. LGBTQ members are twice as likely to suffer from a mental disorder and 2-3 times more likely to attempt suicide.

If you or your partner is suffering, get help before it is too late. In any given year, 60% of people with mental illness don't get the help they need.

## Surviving the 3 D's: Death

I was tangled up in my transformation, pushing ever forward, when death came creeping at my door, unexpectedly, in the middle of one night.

It was June in 2000 when I got a knock at my front door. It was a police officer. He instructed me to call my parents right away!

They had no other way to reach me. At the time, they didn't know my address or phone number. My sister did the mediating.

But this was an emergency. I dressed and flew out the door, because I did not have a home phone. I called my parents' house, and my brother Peter answered. He told me that our other brother Bobby, age twenty-nine, had been killed in a car accident.

Ironically, Linda was at my house that very night. She stayed for days and helped me mourn my brother's death. She held me tight and gave me energy. We lit a stick of jasmine and found a way to a tearful meditation.

Despite five years between us, Bobby and I were closest growing up. He was my little brother. He was a gem to me.

We loved the outdoors. Riding our bikes around our small town gave us a freedom to explore. We jumped in ditches to catch crawdads. We dug for worms to go fishing. We battled the neighborhood kids in kickball.

We had spent a lot of time together.

I once convinced him that we could run away and join the circus if we could find a trick that was risky enough. I talked him into riding his bike off the carport. After a complete failure, his little high-pitched voice he said, "Sister, I don't think this is a good trick!"

The first time I saw Bobby high he was twelve. He worked in a printing company for a few hours after school, a couple days a week. I went to pick him up, and he was stoned. I could smell an odor on his clothing. He high-jumped over the bushes and ran down the street like he was Superman. He had been huffing paint thinner in the back of the shop. I told my parents about my fears regarding his intoxication. But I left home at seventeen, so I don't know how they addressed the situation with him.

He struggled with drug abuse most of his teenage years. He dropped out of high school and moved into a house with older guy at the age of sixteen.

One night, on a long country road, I took out a five-pound pipe wrench that I had hid under the seat of the car. I whaled it around, cursing like mad lady. I confronted him, and thereby, my worst fears. Bobby got out, and I approached him like lioness protecting her cub—unyielding. Exhausted, I swung at him one last time, barely missing his forehead. In my rage, I jumped back into my car and left him standing, perilous, on the old country dirt road. I had literally saved his life.

My outburst came from discovering that he sexually abused one of my daughters. I was shocked, enraged, disbelieving and guilty. I thought by ending the secrecy, it would help heal my family. My parents did not believe the story. Tension rose and loyalties were broken. This began my isolation from my nuclear family.

It was important for me to keep my children safe, so Bobby was not allowed in my house anymore. I wanted my daughter to know that I believed and supported her. She still suffers today from this trauma.

That's one of many reasons I became estranged from my parents.

We did not file charges. To this day, I regret not addressing this with the local police department. It may have changed several lives and ended the secrecy forever.

Bobby was homeless most of the time. When he did find work, he was hard worker. He loved praise. He moved here and there with relatives and stayed off and on in shelters. I know he loved our family. He was protective, capable, strong, and had a half smile. Bobby was a jokester. I know he loved God. People in our town helped him when we were not able to do so. I know he ate food at the mission house on regular basis.

He tried sobriety, and we tried intervention but neither of us had real success.

He lived in an abandoned trailer on the bad side of town.

I would go to check on him couple times a month. He had no utilities and ate fast food or camp-style cooking. It was hard being around an addict who stole and lied just to get to his next high. Several times, I showed up unannounced to find him in a daze, slurring his words and with a chemical smell on him. He had paint stains on his hands and face. He would flail around and yell and beat the walls. I don't know if he even recognized me as his sister. Though I had many reasons why he could not stay at my house, I felt our family should have tried harder.

In 1998, I got letter from one of his past girlfriends telling me that Bobby had fathered a child. The child's name was Christopher Thomas. I met with her and this little, curly blonde-haired toddler. There was no doubt this little guy was my brother's offspring. We both told Bobby. He doubted Christopher was his child. A couple years later, the DNA test proved him wrong. My brother was ordered to pay child support. Today, Christopher has his own struggles in his life. Addiction is a family disease. If not careful and kept in check, it will destroy all things in its path.

Bobby never had trouble meeting women. He was handsome and charming. Then he met a woman named Katrinka, and they began a relationship. I hoped she knew about his drug use. He told me on one visit to his abandoned trailer that he was moving to Plano, Texas.

On another visit, he was sober. Bobby cried and trembled as he hesitated to speak out loud. He said he wanted to change but feared failure. I put my arm around his shoulder gave him a big squeeze that only a sister can give, and we wept together. I said to him that you don't recover from an addiction by stopping the drug. You recover by creating a new life, in which it is easier not to use. He expressed a fear that he was unlovable and weak. He told me of enormous guilt and shame. We talked about recovery and coping skills for a few minutes. With his unwarranted smile and laughter, he changed the subject to moving. I have reflected many times on this conversation.

My brother struggled with his disease. He was a drug addict. I often wondered if he was hiding his own mental illness with substance abuse.

I visited Plano, Texas, once or twice. He lived there off and on for about three years. His girlfriend gave birth to their son Seth on May 5, 2000.

He died in June 2000 while making "a run" for alcohol. Seth was only one month old.

Bobby lost control of the car and smashed into a tree. He had not been wearing his seat belt and broke his neck instantly. I've been told by the person he was living with that he was not sober.

I never took part in the family meetings about his addiction. I did not want to see my parents.

We all knew about it. Most of us practiced tough love. The sad thing is that this heartbreaking story of addiction has become run-of-the-mill these days.

The pain and guilt we all share is extraordinary.

The day after the news of his death, I called my sister and told her that I did not want to go to the funeral. Our family's dysfunction was very raw at this time. My siblings drove to my house and begged me to come. They knew I needed to be there to say one final goodbye.

The funeral was average. The minister spoke about Bobby's life. They played some of his favorite songs. Then shock set in. I was in disbelief. Inside his casket, I saw a brown-headed, mischievous, little five-year-old boy, not the tattooed, hard-shelled adult man. Bobby was laid to rest outside of a small Oklahoma town in a cemetery.

My heart emptied its sorrow as my eyes dripped continuously for days.

But in his death there was a hidden power that no one truly knew. My brother's death had caused a ripple. In God's grace and abiding love, there is purpose. Bobby's death inspired me to reconnect with my parents. A bridge was built. My mother and father started to accept their adult children. They began to connect in new ways that were unfamiliar. My sister was also very engaged with this process.

I believe that God's holy hand was directing them to reach

out and connect with us. This unbelievable move made me revere my spiritual growth. It was our hands that accepted the request.

I am grateful that Bobby's life was not in vain. Our family's love for him will never end. ***And I'm honoring him by pursuing my dreams and living a happy, healthy life.***

Recovering is possible. A family can receive healing. Forgiveness is a powerful truth.

Too frequently, people with mental illness try to self-medicate by turning to alcohol or drugs. This compounds the problem instead of solving it.

Alcohol, in particular, is a depressant, which can exasperate feelings of hopelessness, despair, loneliness, helplessness, etc. Drugs and alcohol are also contributing factors in some suicide cases. In fact, 90% of successful suicides have an underlying mental illness. Depending on the mental illness, between 5 and 30% of sufferers may have co-morbid alcoholism or other problems.

According to the Centers for Disease Control and Prevention (CDC), more than 80,000 people die each year due to a situation related to excessive alcohol use. The CDC also notes that approximately 87 people in America die each day due to an accidental drug overdose. Substance abuse is a big problem in society, which is why most 12-step programs cater to individuals who abuse drugs or alcohol. These 12-step substance abuse rehab centers welcome individuals of all ages as well, so don't ever feel like you are too young or too old to get help.

Don't ever give up, even when you have every reason to do so.

## Surviving the 3 D's: Disease

My disease is called *neutrophilic dermatoses,* a.k.a. Sweet's disease. It is a rare disorder.

In 2011, I spent fifteen days in the hospital and several months off work. I was admitted to the emergency room on August 25th because of a high fever, a skin lesion, and tachycardia.

The doctor suspected severe cellulitis and admitted me to the hospital to stabilize my condition. But my health did not improve after much effort and showed no signs of getting better, despite the PICC line administering high doses of antibiotics and morphine. Friends and family drifted in and out of my hospital room bringing flowers, food and words of encouragement.

One doctor finally performed a biopsy of my skin lesion and determined that the cause of the illness was Sweet's Syndrome (SS).

This is when the team of doctors realized that their expertise was not adequate to treat my condition.

I was transported by ambulance to Oklahoma University Medical Center, seventy-five miles from my home.

The sweats from the fever kept me soaked. I was constantly changing my nightgown. The best way to describe the pain is being burned with a cigarette on different parts of your body. I felt the pain in my joints, bowels and stomach. It was excruciating. I would tremble, wrap my arms around myself, and rock side to side uncontrollably.

This was real. This was a traumatic assault on my body and mind. The nights were unending.

The *prednisone* gave me insomnia. My body and mind would not tolerate sleep. My thoughts raged with negative images bouncing to and fro. I had a constant fear of dying.

The room smelled of urine and death. The odor spun around the room constantly, overwhelming me the minute my eyes closed in the darkness. I was powerless to stop it.

I could hear other patients squealing in pain in rooms close to mine.

My room was quite small, like a camper of sorts. The nurses seemed to take an interest in my situation and offered a smile, a joke and a nice reassuring touch on my arm. This was such a contrast from my experience in a mental health unit. No one came to visit or to empathize with my mental health crisis.

There had been no casseroles from neighbors. No flowers during my hospital stay. I had felt invisible, like I did not matter.

But now, everyone was concerned with my condition. Even the interns asked questions and wanted to capture this rare disease on camera. They took turns snapping photos of the moon-shaped puss pocket the size of a soccer ball on my leg. They said the opportunity might come once in their lifetimes.

There is a time for everything. Hardships and stress are only a season. Change is constant. This, too, shall pass. I repeated these things to myself daily.

Stress wreaks havoc on the mind and body. Until recently, it has not been clear exactly how stress influences disease and health. Now researchers have found that chronic psychological stress is associated with the body losing its ability to regulate the inflammatory response.

People with mental illness have an increased risk of suffering from chronic medical conditions. US adults living with a serious mental disorder die on average 25 years earlier than their mentally healthy counterparts *due to treatable medical conditions!* Don't let your mental health prevent you from getting necessary medical care. You need to take care of both your body and your mind.

It is estimated that $193.2 billion dollars of earnings were lost over the past year due to mental conditions.

In the next section, I will open up my toolkit for those willing to learn how to manage mental health in a positive, affirming manner. What is in your tool box?

## Journaling Questions:

1. What are my tipping points?

2. Do I help others?

3. Do I live honestly?

4. Am I living with a mask?

_____

_____

_____

_____

_____

_____

_____

_____

_____

_____

5. What is my potential?

_____

_____

_____

_____

_____

_____

_____

_____

_____

_____

6. Do I connect with people?

_____

_____

_____

_____

_____

_____

_____

_____

_____

_____

7. Do I get professional help when I need it?

_____
_____
_____
_____
_____
_____
_____
_____

8. Do I feel weak and unlovable?

_____
_____
_____
_____
_____
_____
_____
_____

9. Does my life resemble those in this book?

_____
_____
_____
_____
_____
_____
_____
_____

10. How do I handle stressors?

_____
_____
_____
_____
_____
_____
_____
_____

# Discharge

I had a daily sheet on which I would mark an X if I took my medication. It was difficult to remember much.

Sometimes my hands failed me. Writing words was strenuous. I couldn't process spelling. I would lift a pen but just stare into space. I could not remember words.

My body had endured a tremendous ordeal.

But, even with an unmerciful war being waged in my brain, there was still resilience in my armor. I continued to stumble towards healing.

I tried to make a simple list, but it would only intensify the struggle. Then the list would disappear. And this infuriated me because I had worked so hard to make the list memorable.

Poor concentration, extreme fatigue, and sleep disturbances were all exacerbated by desperation. Every day was a new challenge and another fight.

I made my nest in the extra room in our house. Soon, the feeling of sickness was in the air. The environment reflected it: medication bottles covered the fold-out t.v. tray. The bed was covered in blue pads, because my blistered body wept puss everywhere. There were pieces of scattered paper everywhere. They were discharge instructions from hospital and lists of prescription side-effects.

An abundance of get well cards were propped up on the nightstand.

There was a portable toilet chair next to my bed because my fatigue prevented me from walking more than a few steps. Bottles of water, Sprite, Ensure and snacks were lined up everywhere within reach, like they were going to the movies.

I was incontinent. The strong scent of urine was sometimes over-powering for visitors. The sheets were changed daily, but the smell never left.

My stability was inside my so-called spirit. I fought and resisted with all my heart. I did not want to die.

There was a small CD player in the corner of my room. Most of the time that was my only solace.

My pain was relentless. I had never remembered feeling so much pain before. And I always thought I had a high tolerance.

Movement hurt the most.

The doctor prescribed fentanyl patches for pain relief. My partner would apply one for me before she went to work, so the pain improved for a couple of hours.

I'll take a moment here to mention my wife, Rhonda. She was and has been my rock of support through my disease, recovery, and everything since then.

We went to junior high school together and used to go out for lunch because she had a car. In 2000, a few months after Bobby died, we reconnected at the DHS where I was filing paperwork for a work-related injury. We exchanged contact information and met for another meal.

A few months later, I thought I was making a grand gesture by offering to empty a drawer in my dresser for her things. Rhonda responded that she had already been keeping her clothes in my closet. And those weren't the only things that had to come out of the closet before our relationship could progress.

After my terrible divorce, I vowed never to get married again. Rhonda and I, however, have had two ceremonies—one in 2003, because she had never had a wedding, and another in 2015 when the state of Oklahoma finally legalized gay marriage.

She's the yin to my yang. We work perfectly together. My children love her. Even my ex-husband's family loves her. It's surprising how many allies you have sometimes.

In the throws of my disease, my joy came at the end of the day when Rhonda got home from work. She would touch my arm and tell me things were going to get better. She wrapped her arms around me and held me tight. She massaged my back with oils.

It was like the warmest blanket of white light delicately placed on a dying soul.

I felt as if my body and brain had both forsaken me, and all I had left was waning courage. When my thoughts were clear, I wondered how to ignite my courage and spirit. I also questioned how I would continue the battle.

I could sense that death was in the vicinity. The medications made my thoughts murky. My brain was malfunctioning and stuck. I was an exhausted mess.

Essence of being was the only thing I had left. My spiritual awakening was waiting on me to call out for comfort. But I was resistant to ask for such help. My body was on the mend. It was a transformation, but I had to find my safe place and allow the process. I was silently holding on to the possibility of healing.

I once imagined what I would do if suddenly, I was full of life again. Energetic and healthy, I would go outdoors more, love more, and help others more. Then I was transported back to reality.

We take for granted the ease with which our bodies work until they stop.

With this disease also comes extreme malaise, coupled with depression. I could not do simple tasks. I could not read, write, or think without a constant battle. I needed help with everything.

The worst pain was when my blistered body had to shower, but aggravated pain also accompanied dressing, eating, even moving. I had extreme mood swings and open wounds like boils that drained.

My anxiety ran high when I was left alone. I felt like I was suffocating.

This is when the dark times consumed parts of me. My mind was filled with a gray haze.

Sometimes I wanted to be left alone. My solitude was the only thing I could control. I refused visitors. I felt useless and withdrawn. Hopeless. I was caught up in a hurricane storm of worthlessness.

It was almost impossible to engage myself in anything but my own self-pity.

I could only stand the searing pain of a shower for a few minutes. My weak body would shake uncontrollably. Then I would wither and collapse.

Sleeping well after bathing was impossible because my blistered body had declared another battle.

It was hard to find the proper treatment in my hometown. I saw doctors that had never even heard of this disease, let alone treated it. I was their best source of information.

I understood that my condition was rare, and there were many obstacles in my treatment plan. But after many months at home, the blisters turned to sores and I started wound care.

I would go in twice a week for debriding. That's when the doctor picked off the scabs one-by-one with his special tool kit. It was 30 to 45 minutes of excruciating pain.

Twice a week for six weeks.

Other parts of the healing process weren't as horrible. My strength began to return. My aura became rooted, just like a tree. Deep breathing and meditation became daily rituals. They also gave me a topical cream to help facilitate my body's recovery.

But my struggles with mental health came back to whisper in my ear each night, like a poltergeist spreading negative energy.

It was real and it was damning.

My adult children came to comfort me. Their warm energies became connected to mine. Their gentle touch played a major role in my emotional, mental and medical recovery. I found reassurance in their love for me. This bonding strengthened the roots of my tree.

They cleaned my wounds, helped with household chores, grocery shopped. If there was a need, they were there.

Several times I was rushed to the emergency room with steroid psychoses. The increased dopamine levels in my brain made me lose sense of reality. I often had delusions and sensory flooding, my mind would not stop. It was a repeat of my mental struggles from earlier in my life. I felt like I was facing my deepest fears.

Again.

I had delusions that someone was poisoning my drinks. It seemed unexplainable. An ambulance came to my house because of a panic attack.

You see, corticosteroids are drugs that mimic cortisol, a hormone produced by the body. Cortisol is known as the stress hormone. Because of the long-term steroid use to treat my body, I had adrenal fatigue.

This was another great challenge. It caused my heart to pound and my blood pressure to become low. My fight/flight/freeze instincts kicked in several times a day. This was a terrifying experience for me and those around me

I really thought this was the end. My body was on red alert. I was running a race with myself and I did not know if I would win.

There was a warm sensation elegantly roaming through me. It felt like the oxygen I was breathing was warm. It tingled and left me in a state of grace. I thought I was experiencing death.

I felt like a child, sitting in my tree house, taking in all the commotion around me and internalizing it into stillness and serenity. I was listening to leaves and feeling the warm energy of the sunlight. I even told my best friend that I could feel the sun in my soul. It must be my time to go.

Then, they hit me with some medication in my I.V. and all the symptoms stopped within days. So the truth was out: it was not a mental break this time. It was a medication problem.

This is when I knew I had to find balance and get back to my daily routine. Sitting quietly every morning meditating for ten or fifteen minutes calmed me and helped me find my center.

Eventually, the days turned into weeks and the weeks into months.

My body began to heal. This was time of great reflection. I slept a lot and prayed for my body and mind to heal.

It was hard for me to walk, because of my joints and all the swelling. But I was able to set a goal and achieve it. I could walk to the end of the driveway and back. Slowly, I also started moving to the living room to watch TV. I was able to bathe myself and to take the few steps to the toilet. This was a giant step in my healing process and in my independence.

I wrote thank you cards.

I began to make firm and precise movements without difficulty. My spirit and my body were finally working in unison.

The parts of our lives we take for granted during healthy times seem to be the most valuable when we're not.

I was still taking lots of medication to manage my symptoms. *Cellcept* 500mg is an immunosuppressive and is used when the immune system attacks the body's own tissues. This medication is typically used to treat cancer, organ transplant, lupus, and rheumatoid arthritis patients. *Lisinopril* was used to manage my blood pressure. *Neurontin* 300mg to manage the nerve pain. *Naproxen* 550mg was for muscle aches and swelling. *Tramadol* 50mg treated the pain. *Elavil* 25mg for depression. *Prednisone* for flares. *Sumatriptan* 25mg to remedy the migraines.

I had a dispenser and a chart to help me remember when and what to take.

T h e *prednisone* high dose still made me emotional and moody.

Meanwhile, I was trying to redefine my purpose. I'd passed a tipping point. I found the courage to accept healing.

It was badge of honor to walk into my own positive energy. To trust life.

I had won this struggle and would live to fight another.

There is a poem in my hallway I read everyday called "Do It Anyway" by Mother Teresa:

*People are often unreasonable, irrational, and self-centered.*
**Forgive them anyway.**

*If you are kind, people may accuse you of selfish, ulterior motives.*
**Be kind anyway.**

*If you are successful, you will win some unfaithful friends and some genuine enemies.* **Succeed anyway.**

*If you are honest and sincere people may deceive you.*

**Be honest and sincere anyway.**

*What you spend years creating, others could destroy overnight.*
**Create anyway.**

*If you find serenity and happiness, some may be jealous.*

**Be happy anyway.**

*The good you do today, will often be forgotten.*

**Do good anyway.**

*Give the best you have, and it will never be enough.*

**Give your best anyway.**

*You see, in the final analysis, it is between you and God.*

**It was never between you and them anyway.**

When I was in this humble and hopeless place in my life, someone gave me a copy of *Mother Teresa* by Navin Chawla. Navin is Hindu, but refers to himself as "near atheist," and who better to write a biography than a skeptic? He writes of the facts, which include miracles that occur every day. Mother Teresa herself tells him about these miracles, "If you pray, you will see them." Mother Teresa did what she cared about the most, helping people in need.

**Journaling Questions:**

1. How much energy do I spend on past regrets?

2. How much energy do I use on resentment towards others?

3. How much tension do I carry with me?

4. How does stress and trauma affect my health?

5. How full is my emotional duffle bag that I carry with me everywhere?

_____
_____
_____
_____
_____
_____
_____
_____
_____
_____

6. Who will care for me in my time of need?

_____
_____
_____
_____
_____
_____
_____
_____
_____

7. What am I avoiding or escaping right now because I am afraid?

_____
_____
_____
_____
_____
_____
_____
_____
_____

8. What painful experiences from childhood haunt me and taught me to be afraid?

_____
_____
_____
_____
_____
_____
_____
_____
_____
_____

9. What kind of irrational fears invade my mind?

_____
_____
_____
_____
_____
_____
_____
_____
_____
_____

10. What is one negative belief I have about myself?

_____
_____
_____
_____
_____
_____
_____
_____
_____

# Back to the Workforce

I knew that eventually I would have to return to work. This was my greatest fear. I was scared of what people would say. I was petrified of the rhythm of life in the workforce.

Three months after this ordeal started, I was permitted to return to work part-time.

On the first day back, I discovered that my entire office had been moved to another building. It was in a brick building with lots of parking and no stairs.

My office was in the back corridor. It had no windows. They delivered my furniture and computer, and I started unloading boxes. I was worn out after only an hour.

I took it easy in order to last a few more hours. I needed to get set up and fulfill these new work arrangements. Work meant maintaining my medical insurance.

Fortunately, it was the week of Thanksgiving, so there was a break before I had to return again. I mustered up a belief that this was another tribulation I could survive.

I filed my Family and Medical Leave Act (FMLA) paperwork. My doctor told me that my illness was chronic. While the condition could be managed, it was also recurrent.

I would have to learn to live my life differently. I would require extra breaks. I couldn't climb stairs. There were limitations on how long I could stand and a slew of other restrictions and recommendations. This was my new ordinary.

Eventually, I found my cadence at work.

I would work entering data and filing reports, not unlike any other general office worker. My concentration was still limited, and I sometimes felt a disconnect when processing information.

There was a program at work where other colleagues could donate their leave to anyone in need. My coworkers donated loads of leave time so I could stay on the payroll and still receive a paycheck.

So I had insurance and a paycheck.

I appreciated their kindness. It kept me afloat. If not for their generosity, I would have been homeless, jobless, insurance-less and very, very ill.

This is when the gentle light of God's grace was revealed to me again. Being alone is impossible in a world occupied by angels. I knew I was blessed.

One of my favorite quotes is from Alice Morse Earle: Every day may not be good, but there's something good in every day.

There is gratitude and grace in the midst of every storm. You just have to be willing to look for it.

And this is coming from a hard-working, mother-of-four who had only just graduated from college a few months ago at age forty-five. I started attending Northwestern Oklahoma State University back in 2008 and finished in 2011, right before being diagnosed with Sweet's. On my sick bed, I worried that I would never be able to use the degree in business administration that I had worked so hard for.

Now, I was determined to retain my employment. The word "persevere" was taped on my monitor. I would not accept failure.

Again, I took stock of my mental health issues. I needed to regroup and to design a way that would let me successfully reenter the working world.

I had to rediscover my friends and my enemies. I learned who lifted me up and who stole my energy. I cleaned house, so to speak.

My inner circle of friends were strong players in my recovery. Every foot forward was met with loving care and kindness. When I reached a goal, my teammates helped me celebrate. My foundation had been built through years of hard work, but now I was stumbling on the blocks that had once held me steadfast.

I began fighting the feelings of inadequacy, especially at work. Our jobs are ingrained as part of our identities. I was shaken to the core. But my friends were there to pick up the stones and to help me rebuild. They showed up and helped me collect the pieces of my life.

At times, I could sense stability. I had to trust this process. After the loss of something, we have an opportunity to reinvent ourselves.

I was fired a year and a half after returning to work. During my struggle to heal, both mentally and physically, I got a letter in the mail. It notified me that employment had been terminated due to an inability to perform the duties of my position. Thus, my life story of survival continued.

There is a lot of silver lining to be found in change. The things I thought were out of my reach suddenly became my passion. I was finding my way again and my true identity that I had hidden away.

Be patient. Change takes time. Train yourself in mindfulness. Now my mind is open to new visions. I expand my awareness of my true self.

When you feel paralyzed, devastated, and spinning out of control, remember we all feel this at times in our lives. It is difficult to see hope in the bigger picture. Just remember that pain is inevitable and suffering is optional.

◆◆◆◆

**Journaling Questions:**

1. Do/should I disclose mental illness in the workplace?

2. Can concealing illness raise the stressors at my workplace?

_____
_____
_____
_____
_____
_____
_____

3. How can I (or we) change the discrimination and stigma related to mental illness?

_____
_____
_____
_____
_____
_____
_____

4. Can I ask for reasonable accommodations if I have a mental disorder?

_____
_____
_____
_____
_____
_____
_____

5. When was a time that I was vulnerable and lost at my job?

_____
_____
_____
_____
_____
_____
_____

# Part 2 – The Recovery

## The Plan

This toolkit is the crux of the healing process. It is written for individuals suffering from mental disorders but can also be utilized by those helping them. These seven steps will guide you through the process of working through any problem. The guidelines stretch from the beginning to the end, and there are no limits to the scope of this tool. You can use it for your overall mental healthcare plan, or you can use it to cope with a bad day. I am happy to tell you that there are ways to manage and maintain a healthier lifestyle.

There are several reasons for beginning a life change. This is the time for preparation. Check all of the following that apply to you:

◊ I am supporting someone in making healthy choices.

◊ I am looking for opportunities to increase the diversity in a working plan.

◊ I want to review new tools to help prevent stagnation.

◊ I want to improve my knowledge of understanding different struggles.

◊ I am inspired to do better and to be accountable.

◊ I want to erase differences, misunderstandings and stigma.

◊ I want to provide more value to individuals who live with mental health issues.

◊ I want to invest in my own growth and development.

◊ I want to improve my overall motivation and to rejuvenate others who are willing to change.

◊ I want to better serve individuals and their support systems.

◊ I want to identify a network of resources.

◊ I want to build relationships and trust.

◊ I want equal treatment for all within employment.

◊ I want to help build a community that embraces the dignity of all its citizens.

# Step One: Recognition – Name the Disorder

In general, this step involves beginning to find treatment and help.

Acknowledge that your situation may be beyond your control, and that you will not be able to solve it on your own. Learn to say *"I need help."*

Start by calling your doctor and/or mental health practitioner and telling him or her what is going on with you.

Call a friend or tell a co-worker.

Mental illness is a disease in the brain and must be treated as such. It is not so different from a fracture or infection.

It can be helpful to name the disorder (such as bipolar, chronic depression, etc.) or to have a proper diagnosis. You might ask why you need to know these details about your disorder. The answer is that knowledge is power. Knowing what you're up against will help you overcome it.

Decide how you will educate yourself, both about your diagnosis and about suggested solutions. This is a great way to get started and will encourage your productivity for the rest of this process. Also identify what your fears are and what obstacles you may encounter along the way. For example: *I am sometimes my greatest obstacle. I feel that my family and friends expect me to behave in a certain way and that I have to live up to their expectations. I'm afraid of change.*

These transformations require education and dedication. This will provide you with the right information, support, and resources to change in the most beneficial way.

If you are reading this book, you may need to transform. The good news is that you already holding an excellent tool in your hands! This entire book is full of resources and advice. When there is something missing, knowledge is power. This is the season for growing.

Others may be telling you to change, but you must be the one to *want* change.

You know there is more to life than where you are right here and now. You might be questioning your purpose in life. Take off your shoes and become grounded for a moment. Feel the earth under your feet.

Really, go outside and do it.

Whatever the reason, it is time to consider a change.

Work with your support team (the people with whom you've chosen to surround yourself and are aware of your situation) to gather up information about your situation or condition.

Everyone must agree to the goal and be willing to invest the time and teamwork in order to achieve success.

Collaboration is very important, both for individuals and the support system. You must be willing to trust and share your thoughts and feelings with each other.

You also need to set goals. Weekly goals can be time-consuming for the individual and the team, but this is the most important component of the task.

Some of the goals may simply be living skills, such as house cleaning, working, and cooking.

Help your team identify these tasks. Make the goals *simple, achievable and measurable* (SAM). Remember this simple abbreviation, SAM. Make sure to add a timeframe for completion. This is the season of preparation.

All team members must participate in the daily goal-setting for this phase to be productive.

There will be fears and resistance along the way. It may feel like a hot sweaty summer day, but remember there is a time for everything. Often times, as soon as you start progressing, you will encounter resistance. There will always be something trying to stop you, or so it may seem.

Remember mental illness can't be cured. However, it can be managed.

I was there once, fearing both failure and success. I had concentration problems. I still fight chronic depression. My biggest obstacle is myself.

You must be able to move out of the way and accept healing.

You must identify your fear and take action in spite of it. It's time for some maturity.

Now is the time to walk steady and slowly in a progressive forward motion.

◆◆◆◆

**Journaling Questions:**

1.  How will I educate myself?

2.  What are my fears?

3. What are some obstacles I may face in the future? (Don't forget to consider your friends, family, job, and even yourself.)

4. Am I willing to be accountable and willing to change?

**5.** What support systems do I have in place now, and how can they work better?

**6.** Do I have a medication treatment plan, and is it working for me?

**7.** What are my goals?

_____
_____
_____
_____
_____
_____
_____
_____
_____
_____
_____
_____
_____
_____
_____

8. Where are the gaps between me and achieving this goal?

_____
_____
_____
_____
_____
_____
_____
_____
_____
_____
_____
_____
_____
_____
_____
_____
_____
_____
_____
_____

**9.** Do I need help?

_____
_____
_____
_____
_____
_____
_____
_____
_____
_____
_____
_____
_____
_____
_____
_____
_____
_____

**10.** Who can I talk to who will understand?

_____
_____
_____
_____
_____
_____
_____
_____
_____
_____
_____
_____
_____
_____

## Step Two: Expansion – Become the Architect of Your Own Destiny

Only begin this step once you have completed the recognition phase and determined the requirements for completing your plan.

This phase involves writing objectives. It also involves team and individual support.

First, create learning objectives. A *learning objective* is a statement of what you will be able to do once you have completed your goal. Make the objectives concise, understandable, and achievable.

Example: *I want to learn to pay my bills. I will learn about one utility bill a month. I will take money to the office and pay the bill. I will organize the receipts in a folder. I will check off the bill on list after it is paid. The goal will be evaluated by a parent or custodian.*

Notice that this example uses the when/where/how approach; whenever possible, include a time (when), a location (where), and a means (how) in your learning objectives.

This is very simple task to start. This example will build confidence and social skills.

Another example: *I will spend relaxed and quiet time by myself. I will learn to relax in quiet space.* When/Where/How: *I will set aside a block of time. I will turn off all electronics. I will take three deep breaths, inhaling as if I'm smelling a rose, exhaling as if I am blowing out a candle. I will close my eyes and concentrate on my breathing. I will feel my own warm, positive energy.*

I include a third example here because it's often critical for recovery: *I will take my medication as prescribed by my doctor. I will use a checklist or weekly pill box. A guardian, trusted friend, or other member of my team will hold me accountable by verifying my checklist, calling me daily, asking about my medication habits, etc.*

Other examples of learning objectives: keep a journal; read daily affirmations; set aside time for something you enjoy; seek help when you need it; call your family and friends; examine your triggers; learn to express anger responsibly; take walks; become more aware of your feelings; improve your communication; avoid alcohol or drugs; learn to forgive yourself or others.

Once you have established your learning objectives, use your own compass to map the course. Remember, SAM: make goals simple, achievable, and measurable. Add a timeline if it would help.

Think of the learning objectives as your roadmap to success and you are the navigator. Remember there is time to be born, time to die, time to plant and time to harvest. Remember what season of life you are in. Reflections and affirmations are needed to balance your recovery. Move forward slowly but steadily.

It may feel fake or foreign at first. Try to work on your goals anyway. It will be training for your mind. Changes do not happen overnight. It takes lots of practice and patience. Psychologically speaking, it takes twenty-one days to form a new habit.

Think of yourself as a butterfly. You are in the caterpillar stage eating lots of information. Learn how to live with mental illness. This is your transformation stage. Think of spring the time for blooming. There is a time for everything. Don't try to manage it. Let it flow naturally.

The pupa stage could be your tipping point. Take some time to rest and find your internal compass. Think of traveling out of town with no map or g.p.s., no Google or Siri. Often times this is how we live our lives. No roadmap or direction. Make a vision board or draw out a plan of where you are going in this healing journey.

Learn to love and accept yourself. Then, and only then, will you emerge a beautiful butterfly with wings for travel.

Create a vision board. Track your personal growth by making a chart. Deepen your connection with the Divine (whatever that may mean to you). Explore your inner-self through relaxation and meditation.

Talk to others about your milestones. Spend time thinking creatively. Start journal about your changes and your goals. Plan your own wellness.

With every good plan, there must be a start date. Discuss the dates with your team.

Begin.

◆◆◆◆

**Tasks:**

1. Continue journaling.

2. Direct your creative energies into something positive.

3. Draw your own compass:

4. Draw what your transformation will look like:

5. Create a vision board or a chart of your own destiny:

# Step Three: Wellness Plan – Manage Crises

Individuals do better with change if they know when and how things are going to change.

Let the people around you know that you are investing time and energy into achieving a balanced, healthier life. Now that you are a butterfly with wings to travel, there may still be a need for intervention. That's okay.

Our lives are always changing and certain circumstances can trigger us: death, trauma, stress, and divorce are a few examples we've already discussed.

When living with mental illness, the road may not be easy. However, you can find a way to thrive by planning ahead. Remember mental illness cannot be cured, but it can be managed.

Times of crisis may occur less and less over time. However, you still need a preparedness plan. This is the awakening stage.

To escape your prison of self-doubt, you will need a plan to construct your own destiny. You are your own architect.

Make sure everyone close to you knows the plan. Include phone numbers, crisis hotlines, and doctors in high-traffic areas. Make sure a list of your medications and diagnoses are readily available.

Check with your local law enforcement about CIT. Be sure to store your documents in more than one place.

Make sure the wellness plan, as you've written it, is followed by everyone.

**Things to discuss with your team members:**

1.  How much does happiness and mental health mean to you?

    _____
    _____
    _____
    _____
    _____

2. Will you be able to support me in the long haul?

_____
_____
_____
_____
_____
_____
_____

3. How can using this toolkit and its strategies improve your life?

_____
_____
_____
_____
_____
_____
_____

4. How can you expand that impact to your family and community?

_____
_____
_____
_____
_____
_____
_____

5. In the event of a crises, how will everyone proceed?

_____
_____
_____
_____
_____
_____
_____

You should also talk about how your life has been affected by your mental condition. Examine yourself to see if you are lying to yourself or others about your illness. Acknowledge if you use alcohol or drugs to cover up your illness.

It can also be helpful to talk about any negative feelings you may have about your illness. Feeling shame and guilt is common.

Have an accountability plan. Find someone who will hold you accountable for your actions. Discuss if your illness affects you or others financially. If you can, open about your lowest feelings and experiences and express that you never want to be there again.

Finally, find allies or support groups or talk to your clergy.

It will also be necessary to forgive yourself for any past transgressions. You have to forgive yourself before you can accept forgiveness from others.

Practice living a manageable life. Speak it. Read it. Hear it. Taste it. Feel it every day. Soon your body and mind will get into the routine of your new changes. Life is a series of waves that have a certain rhythm. This rhythm is important to embrace and cooperate with. Similarly to learning an instrument or developing another talent, you have to practice.

It is not an easy process. It is okay not to be alright all of the time. Everything changes, good things, bad things, satisfying and unsatisfying... All are constantly flowing.

These empowering tools that can be arranged to fit any needs. Mental illness has a spectrum, from mild to moderate and severe. If you need to start with one goal a day or write a month of goals, it's your choice. You are the architect and you design your own plan. Do things your way. Get started as soon as possible!

Example: *My wellness plan consists of daily routines, such as eating healthy meals, doing yoga, meditating, helping others, and writing.* I stick with my wellness plan. I found my roadmap.

I've slowly carved out a life that works for me. Life is art! We're all on a journey, but our paths are unique to us.

I also learned to empty my mind of all the old recordings and false purposes that I had been taught. There is a beginning and ending to everything. You must let go of past regrets to make better choices. Just as you let go of your mistakes, you must let go of others' mistakes. Because life is a process, we should always be doing *something*.

Once, I was reading a great mystery novel with the women of my local book club. I loved it from the beginning. This was unusual because I had not previously enjoyed mysteries. The book took twists and turns. Both good and bad characters surprised me. The suspense ratcheted up chapter after chapter. I did not want the story to end. The book developed vivid, lovable personalities.

As I was nearing the end of the book, an emptiness started to grab a hold of me. You see, emptiness is a process, too. It means that something is finishing while something else is beginning. This was a great lesson in mindfulness to me. Changes are what make life interesting.

Open yourself to opportunities and let the process begin. It helps to know how emotions, thoughts and attitude affect your energy. Also, soon you will begin to realize that stress has negative impacts on your energy levels.

As I began to fulfill my purpose, I could see my wellness plan working. I knew I would still experience times of stress, however, I felt better armed to handle these stressful situations.

As you begin your wellness plan, remember mental health is your responsibility. Identify your triggers and early warning signs, and talk about your crisis plan. You are in charge of your own recovery.

While you are working towards wellness, remember to thank those supporters around you and know that you are also helping other in your existence.

## Step Four: Implementation – Put Your Plan into Action

Put your plan into action. This step is the simplest, but it can also take the longest.

Every day is a different opportunity for choices. Life presents us with new challenges every day. Now that have made your wellness plan, put it into action and let yourself morph into a beautiful butterfly. Begin to see your transformation in you reflection. You have to be able to move forward. See it. Hear it. Speak it. Think it. Feel it. Then breathe and do it again.

There will be setbacks and failures. It may feel like everything and everyone is pushing against you. Roadblocks are not a part of the plan, however, they're bound to be there. Take a break if you need one, but don't give up.

Just as there will be problems, there will also be times of solace and joy as you achieve small victories. The ability to organize and design your own plan will give you strength and assurance in yourself.

It's like your own GPS: you know the coordinates, so you can get there if you're willing to make the necessary changes.

Expect to confront your fears over the process of implementation. You can overcome them.

Healing changes your universe. People will begin to take notice of your changes. Your friends and family may struggle with accepting this change. They may have been taking care of your needs for a long time, and they will have their own fears. Show them patience and respect as they learn to let go.

Each step to independence is a stone in a foundation of trust. Let them know you have developed a plan. There may be some challenges that they can still help you with. Make a list and share it with them.

Share your victories and keep them informed as to where you are within your wellness plan. Slow and steady communication will help others adjust to your transformation. As they see you grow to your true potential, they will learn to celebrate with you. Surround yourself with hopeful people. Hope is contagious!

Seize the moment. Believe you're a part of something bigger than yourself. It's okay to dream big.

Take the state of Oklahoma (where I have lived my entire life) for example: Its story is one of hope, resiliency, rebirth and renewal.

The story starts with the Trail of Tears. In the 1830's, Andrew Jackson forced the Cherokee Indian nation to give up their lands east of the Mississippi and migrate to what is today known as Oklahoma. The Cherokee people named it the Trail of Tears because of its devastating effect on their people. One fourth of the people traveling on the trail died.

The journey was approximately one thousand miles. These wounds ran deeply and traumatically. There was a deep violation of humankind and a sense of hopelessness along the trail.

But these indigenous people survived against all odds.

There are not many places you can go in Oklahoma and not see the compassion and tenderness of the Cherokee people. Each step forward was hope for the new generation. There are statues, museums, and revivals of traditions and cultural renewal. In fact, Oklahoma's name comes from two Choctaw words meaning *red people*.

A Native American stands tall on our state capitol building.

Every summer in Oklahoma, there are American Indian pow-wow festivals, surrounding our communities with cultural elements. These celebrations bring dance, song, friendship, and competition. These sacred traditions live on in a circle of unity. Our fellow Oklahomans chose to rise up beyond their traumas and become an Indian nation again. This is a reminder of how healing changes the universe. Oklahoma has a strong spirit because of our shared history and culture.

This is just one example of how, over a long period of time, all resistance, adversaries and obstacles can be overcome. Finding a solution isn't always easy. The good news is that you have a resource of information in your hands right now.

# Step Five: Evaluation – Determine the Benefits

After the first couple of months on your new wellness plan, evaluate your progress. Decide which things worked and which didn't. Let your internal compass be your guide. Remember this is your road and your map.

Tweak your plan in the way that best fits your needs. For example, I chose to use a spread sheet so I could check off the goals I accomplished daily. My achievements helped to build a foundation where I could live a healthier lifestyle.

Evaluation offers you a way to determine if your wellness plan is working.

◆◆◆◆

## Journaling Questions:

1. Did I get the results I was expecting?

_____
_____
_____
_____
_____
_____
_____
_____
_____
_____

2. Did I achieve the positive changes I wanted?

_____
_____
_____
_____
_____
_____
_____
_____
_____
_____

3.  What other changes need to be made?

    _____
    _____
    _____
    _____
    _____
    _____
    _____
    _____
    _____
    _____

4.  What strategies worked?

    _____
    _____
    _____
    _____
    _____
    _____
    _____
    _____
    _____
    _____

5.  How will I continue to monitor my mental health?

    _____
    _____
    _____
    _____
    _____
    _____
    _____
    _____
    _____
    _____

6. Did I achieve physical, social and emotional well-being?

_____
_____
_____
_____
_____
_____
_____
_____
_____
_____
_____
_____

7. Did I prioritize my goals in order of importance?

_____
_____
_____
_____
_____
_____
_____
_____
_____
_____
_____

8. Did I gain friends and build relationships during this time?

_____
_____
_____
_____
_____
_____
_____
_____

9. Am I building my true life path?

_____

_____

_____

_____

_____

_____

_____

_____

_____

_____

_____

_____

_____

_____

_____

10. What do I think when I look in the mirror?

_____

_____

_____

_____

_____

_____

_____

_____

_____

_____

_____

_____

_____

_____

_____

Remember, success varies greatly for each individual.

# Step Six: Education – Educate Yourself and Others

I talked about struggle and recovery. I described how to recognize mental health issues. I designed and developed a plan to be held accountable on the road to success. I've realized that mental health can be managed and recovery is possible. Now that my life was less chaotic, a need for companionship arose.

So my continued education concerned relationships and sex. (Finally, the good stuff!)

Your education might look different. For now, I want to share with you what I learned.

Most people want to have a partner to connect with intimately and emotionally. Every day, we see couples together at coffee shops, book stores, and benches on the courthouse lawn. People hold hands walking down the street. Internet dating is now the normal. Commercials are full of relationship enthusiasm. It can sometimes make you feel like you're the only single person in the world.

Satisfying a need for intimate relationships is highly relevant to overall health and mental wellbeing for everyone. People need love and companionship. It's a part of being human.

Remember how you felt the first time you fell in love? Sometimes, we are so caught up in our disorders and problems that we forget the good stuff. We become accustomed to being alone because we are so withdrawn from the world. We connect with no one because it is easier than explaining why we act the way we do.

One-night stands are common among people with mental health struggles.

You may have to overcome past trauma in order to move forward with relationships.

As you start your path to healing, things begin to change. Difficult situation become less common, and your confidence will start to improve. This allows you to truly believe that you are loveable and deserve a companion.

There is, of course, a degree of anxiety and complexity in building a healthy relationship with someone. And while there are challenges, the rewards are enormous. I have been in a long-term, loving relationship for fifteen years. This has been a test of my wits and my need to feel loved and appreciated. I often questioned my sanity for getting into another relationship after a failed marriage. But I'm so glad I took another chance for love. Here are some of the things I struggled with and learned about.

1. Anger can be a side effect of medication.

2. Medication also affects libido, orgasm, and erection.

3. Feeling undesirable is common among people with low self-esteem and mental illness.

4. It's a challenge to feel "good enough."

5. Both partners have a say in what happens during sexual intimacy.

6. Communication is key.

7. When sexually active, there is a risk of STDs.

8. Finding a good partner and establishing a healthy relationship is difficult.

Fortunately, the good outweighs the bad by far. I've learned to love another human being.

According to Substance Abuse and Mental Health Services Administration (SAMHSA), people that maintain healthy relationships have higher rates of recovery.

Sexual expression is part of my happiness. Love has made me a better person. Now would be a good time to thank my partner, Rhonda, for her unending love and concern for my wellbeing.

Here is another list of things we learned together:

- Compromise
- Communication
- Affection
- Acceptance
- Trust
- Support
- Financial Responsibility
- Love
- Respect

◆ Travel  ◆ Endless benefits

◆ Forgiveness

Never expect someone to be your everything. This is a recipe for failure. You must have outside interests and friends. Keep your mental health a priority. It is easy to get caught up in a new relationship. If your goal is to find a long-term relationship, start with building a foundation that will support this goal. You may be asking how to do this.

First, start with an assessment of yourself as a candidate for a successful relationship.

◆◆◆◆

**Journaling Questions:**

1. Can I be trusted?

 

 

 

 

 

 

 

 

 

 

 

2. Can I be intimate with someone?

3.  Can I say yes to my needs even if they conflict with others?

_____

_____

_____

_____

_____

_____

_____

_____

4.  Can I leave a situation that is abusive to me?

_____

_____

_____

_____

_____

_____

_____

5.  Can I open my heart?

_____

_____

_____

_____

_____

_____

_____

_____

_____

_____

_____

_____

_____

_____

These are questions from the book *Healing Words and Affirmations for Adult Children of Abusive Parents* by Steven Farmer that I often read during times when I'm struggling. It helps me release the old ways of thinking and feeling.

If you can honestly answer these questions, you may be ready for success in your personal life. Allowing another person and a romantic, loving companionship into your life journey may happen soon. If you can't, then you may have some things to work on. Life is full of journeys, and we never know what opportunities unfold down the road. Just because you are not ready now does not mean that you will never be in a long-term relationship.

While this section has focused on educating yourself about relationships, education can take many other forms. Instead or also, you might research the services covered by your healthcare provider. Invest in finding a psychologist or psychiatrist who is good for you. Remember, this may require some traveling. Don't settle.

Educate yourself about your own strengths and weaknesses. This can help when you continue to plan for your future. Within this realm, it may be necessary to make amends, ask for forgiveness, or even pay back monetary expenses incurred by others.

Your education could be finding and engaging in other creative outlets. Read a book, learn a musical instrument, take a class. These activities keep your mind active and can be new, healthy coping methods for you to discover.

Educate yourself about your physical health. This could include losing weight, cutting back on sugars or processed ingredients, leaning to cook, starting an exercise regime, etc.

Explore different religions, or discover what the Divine means to you.

Be patient. Slow and steady. Take one step at a time.

# Step Seven: Empowerment – Achieve a Greater Sense of Confidence

First, I want to say congratulations for making it this far. Continue your journey. One of my favorite quotes from *Eat, Pray, Love* is "Happiness is not something ready made, it comes from your own actions." This inspires me to be responsible for my own happiness.

Look around your local area and find support groups that can help you network with others and find your own voice. It can be a volunteer or mentor situation. Almost any group can help. Find ways of empowerment. Hope is contagious.

Weight Watchers and Alcoholics Anonymous are good examples of programs that may be in your local area. These programs have been around for a long time and have a high success rate. Example: I recently joined a meditation group at my local gym.

Find a place that understands your condition and is willing to help you network to find others. You can start your own group if there is nothing in your local area. Example: I volunteer at a senior center, helping deliver groceries and transporting seniors to doctor appointments.

Begin a gratitude journal. You might find that you are part of something bigger than yourself. Discover more things that bring you pleasure.

I count my achievements and repeat them to myself, my friends and my family.

I use my journal to help me navigate my path. If I see many blessings in one area, I try to open up to more opportunities by continuing to learn and visualizing my direction.

This is how I came to be an author.

I had a dream! But I had I kept it buried deep inside – almost invisible. I started noticing a pattern in my journaling but I denied it for a long time. Finally, I've opened myself up to the opportunity and, little by little, my dream has become a reality. I had to grow and to overcome a lot of suffering to get here. Believe that you are worthy of a gift, however, and let the healing change your reality.

I was successful in my late college education, learning to love research and write essays. After Peter's near-death experience, I experimented with writing from his perspective. Over and over in my head, however, I heard, *You're not qualified to write a book. You don't have enough skills or knowledge. Your writing won't be any good.* There were minefields of critics inside my own head.

Fortunately, in our local book club, we read *Playing Big* by Tara Mohr. She talks about combining your inner skills and trying to train yourself with daily practices. That book helped me diffuse those minefields which were only holding me back. Mohr also provides ten ways to grow your inner mentor. I practice them constantly and recommend her book to anyone.

Parts of the story you are reading today sat lifeless for years. But they're not anymore.

In my journal, I keep track of dreams, feelings, situations, and most of all, thankfulness. I want to share some entries with you:

*Great Day!!*

*Tama came down to visit from OKC. We went to Misti and Pat's house for a celebration. We had a great dinner and conversation. Karen, a numerologist I have never met before, gave me a reading. I really knew nothing about numerology. It's a mystical science between numbers and events. It also pertains to astrology, I think. She said my numbers: 2-7-9. Her readings were very accurate regarding my journey.*

*I asked Karen if she interpreted dreams. She said she did, so I repeated a dream I had a month before. "I was driving with my grandson Will in the car. We came to a stop light in my town, and there was a black man reading from the Bible in a manner that I recognized as erratic.*

*"He shouted with the Holy Bible in his hand. His tattered clothes and unkempt hair were the first signs. He yelled some verse toward us, and I replied with a derogatory comment.*

*"The light turned green, and I went on my way.*

*"I noticed in the rear-view mirror this man was now riding a bicycle, catching up to me. The faster I went, the faster he went. We finally met at a stop light. He rode up to the driver's door and said that was not a nice thing to say.*

*"Then he was transformed into a shaman with a colorful headdress.*

*"He told me to follow the turtle. Do not forget the turtle! Over and over he said, DO NOT forget the turtle. I felt like a message had been delivered, than an old truth had been rekindled."*

*Karen's interpretation was that the stop light was a crossroads.*

*All the characters were parts of me: I was crazy, I was a child, I was the driver in my own life. I could be a wise thinker, or a practicing healer. I should trust and love myself.*

*And if a turtle shows up in my life, it is time to get connected to my most primal essence.*

*Go within your shell and come out when your ideas are ready to be expressed. It is time to recognize that there is an abundance out there for you. It doesn't have to be gotten quickly and immediately. Take your time and let the natural flow work for you.*

That day I secretly vowed to find my truth. I've also gone on to share the turtle dream with many people, friends, family, even casual acquaintances. They all understand that there was a powerful message in that dream and are inspired to look for deeper meaning in their own lives.

◆◆◆◆

*I think people are in my life for a reason. My story, my lessons, are part of their stories. I was able to lead a project called Burning Spam, sponsored by the Enid LGBT Coalition, at Roman Nose State Park in October of 2015.*

*Burning Spam was created as a life class to help share creativity and find our true potential. We burned the spam of negative thoughts that we received from others and ourselves by fellowship and meditation. The purpose of the retreat is that people* tend to live longer lives that when they surround themselves with healthy behaviors and social relationships. This was a way to find your tribe. We learned to let go of things that no longer served us. We carved out new intentions for our futures.

Thank you guest presenters: Jennifer Ippolito & Karen Harris of Healing States 365 and Rev. Jeni Markham Clewell. I can't thank you enough for your service to our community. This was an amazing weekend. The workshop was designed to be a way to celebrate diversity in our community by combining mind, body and spirit. It was to promote healthy behaviors and social relationships. This was time for transformation.

On Saturday morning, we were part of a smudging ceremony with sage. This spiritual cleansing helps combat negative energy and helps you start anew. The leaders took the dried sage and an owl feather. They lit the sage and smoke filled the outside air. The sage is the earth and the smoke is the air. Then they took oils and blessed our foreheads.

We had lots of discussion on letting go of things that no longer serve us. We ate together. We laughed together. We cried together. We shared our stories.

We had a bonfire to burn and to let go of our spam.

The ceremony began with the beating of a drum. We were asked to state our name and invoke our ancestors to the gathering to heal all our wounds. The fire keepers tended to the scared flame. Tobacco and sage were offer to the fire. The drum was passed around, rotating clockwise, neighbor-to-neighbor during the ceremony. We each offered a sacrifice to the flame. We named our intentions of letting go of things that no longer serve us. The coyotes sung for us in the distance. Mother Earth dropped a light rain on our great round. Each individual was directed to use one word they hoped to receive during this retreat. We closed with giving thanks. Then the circle was closed.

I felt the universe and the group become one. The energy was united as it should be in our lives. Our electric current is now plugged in to the great round.

Oneness.

*I am connected to all things, living and nonliving.*

*We were able now to see a vision of our life path.*

*It is strength. There are seasons of sorrow, joy, hardship, and preparation. The one thing that is constant is change. God is always working. I am learning to trust my higher power.*

*I have always known it was there waiting to reveal itself at just the right moment. It is like the tree that I regularly draw. I can't get my mind off this tree. It has seasons in the middle and all these figures round the outside.*

Continuously be open to healing is the key to recovery.

This is my reminder to you that life is always changing.

Today I feel loved and accepted. This is my day, and I paid attention.

How do we find a way for empowerment? According to iempowerself.com, self-empowerment is one of the simplest forms of taking charge of your life. It is a process. Many may know the word empowerment but few really put it into action.

This chapter reveals how to gain knowledge in one's self. The ability to awaken, make needed changes, learn new skills, and activate personal power. The power is in the commitment and dedication to developing yourself.

Repeat your good qualities often. Visualize these qualities by journaling and in silent meditation. Exercise these qualities by putting them into action.

Let go of perfection.

Always remember that the source of happiness lies within.

I often wondered what my core being looked like. Our souls represent our entire element of existence. The soul is the essence of our living selves. If our souls have sounds, what would they be?

I believe this is part of our evolutionary journey. I think love, service, stewardship, connections and expressing creativity are the most important parts of the spirit.

This quote can nicely sum up the essence of a soul:

*You don't have a soul. You are a Soul. You have a body.*
-Walter M. Miller, Jr.

Get out your journal. I challenge you to draw your own spirit.

**Journaling Questions:**

1. Knowledge is power. How can I commit to finding more knowledge?

_____
_____
_____
_____
_____
_____
_____
_____
_____
_____
_____
_____

2. How can I be accountable?

_____
_____
_____
_____
_____
_____
_____
_____
_____
_____
_____
_____
_____
_____

3. How can I be more proactive and less reactive?

_____
_____
_____
_____
_____
_____
_____
_____
_____
_____

4. How do I express self-empowerment?

_____
_____
_____
_____
_____
_____
_____
_____
_____

5. Why do I think I need to be perfect?

_____
_____
_____
_____
_____
_____
_____
_____
_____
_____
_____
_____

6. When will I take action?

_____
_____
_____
_____
_____
_____
_____
_____
_____

7. How do I visualize my healing?

_____
_____
_____
_____
_____
_____
_____
_____
_____

8. Will I start a gratitude journal?

_____
_____
_____
_____
_____

9. Do I have a daily ritual of affirmations?

_____
_____
_____
_____
_____
_____
_____
_____

## 10. Do I believe in my truth?

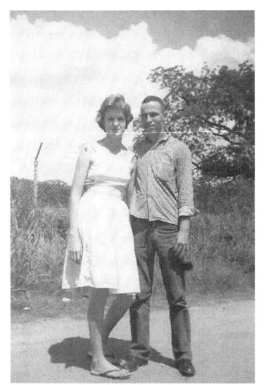

*My parents, shortly before they got married.*

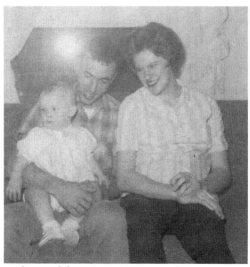

*My parents and my older sister. My mother is pregnant with me.*

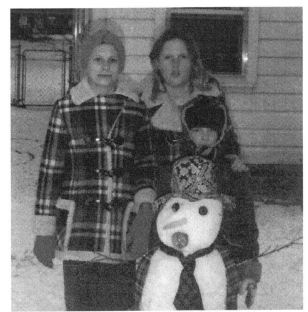

*Cheryl, me, and Bobby.*

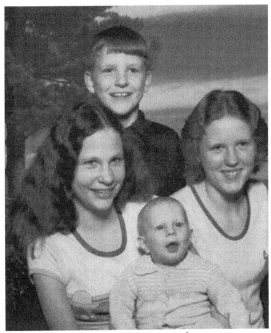

*Just after Peter was born.*

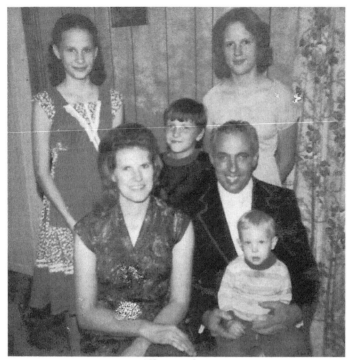

*All six of us.*

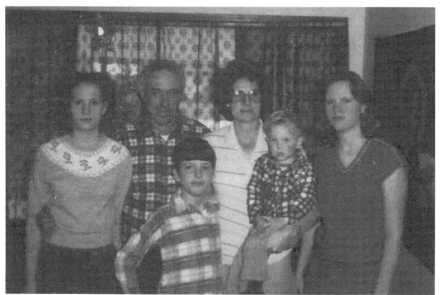

*I was about 17 in this picture.*

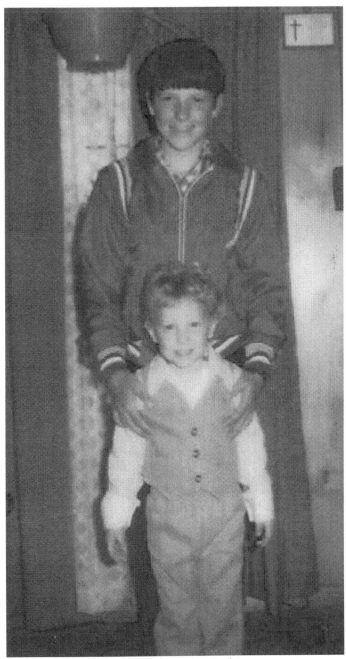

*My brothers, Bobby and Peter.*

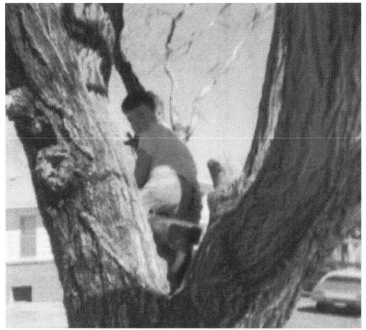

*Bobby in the tree.*

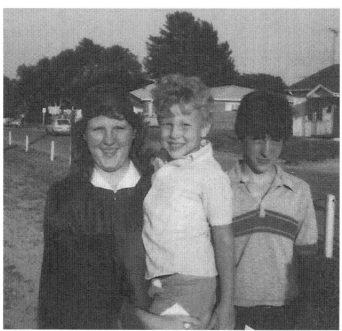

*My high school graduation, a few months after my son was born.*

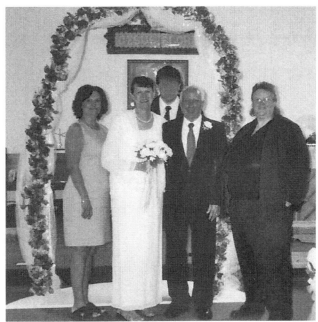

*My parents' 40<sup>th</sup> wedding anniversary, a few years after Bobby died.*

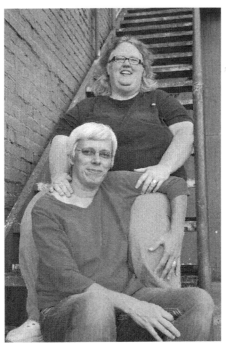

*My engagement photo with my wife, Rhonda.*

# Part 3 – The Healing

# Ending the Silence

To help me stay balanced, I invented a little tag line. I needed something easy to remember and that I could use even when I wasn't thinking clearly.

It goes: Sleep, Nutrition, Activity, People (SNAP).

We will explore these one at a time, starting with sleep.

Sleep plays vital role in good health and wellbeing throughout our lives, according to the U.S. Department of Health and Human Services. Getting enough sleep supports healthy brain function. Strive to get 8 to 10 hours a day. Sleep helps your brain work properly. Depression is now the leading cause of disability, affecting more than 120 million people worldwide. Sleep also plays an important role in your physical health, too, as the body does most of its healing at night.

Regarding nutrition: try to reduce your intake of refined sugars and caffeine. Eat three healthy meals a day. Doing this also improves your heart health. Don't skip meals.

As I am writing this, I realize that it is past lunchtime. I need to follow my own advice and get some nutrition into my body. This was one of the hardest things for me to learn. In the past, unhealthy eating was one of the first signs that I was in crisis. Recognizing this has lead to great benefits.

Remember caffeine can trigger mania and impair sleep. Before making radical changes in your diet consult with your physician.

According to book *The Paleo Cure,* we were never meant to eat the sugar, refined flour and industrial seed oils that are a mainstay in the standard American diet. This may contribute to the 12.7 million strokes annually worldwide. In addition, diabetes and obesity affect over 100 million Americans and 1 billion people across the world. Be mindful of what you put into your body.

The activity part of SNAP means get up an exercise! I have physical limitations, but that is no excuse. I do chair yoga in the morning. People with mental illness are at higher risk for medical illnesses. I notice in the summer if I go outside for a few hours a day and absorb what the sunshine has to offer, I feel better. The warmth gives me energy. The exposure to the sun is thought to increase the brain's release of a hormone called serotonin. This is associated with helping mood boosting and calm and focused feelings. It is that simple.

Exercise helps to improve energy levels, concentration, and sleep, all of which are important for people living with mental illness. Try walking, tai chi, joining a gym, following an exercise video, etc.

The last part of SNAP is people, meaning social relationships.

*Be around people. Go visit the sick or take a class at the local technology school. Join a book club or go to a workshop. Make it a point to leave the house at least once a week to connect with others. Social isolation is a recipe for trouble. Make a list of family members and supportive people in your life. Stay in touch with them regularly. Make social plans. Strengthen your relationship with others by doing fun things.*

Here are some other examples:

◆ Start a card night

◆ Play board games

◆ Organize movie nights

◆ Join a book club

◆ Arrange a potluck dinner

◆ Skype or FaceTime someone you love who lives far away

◆ Join a casual sports team

◆ Accompany other parents who walk and stroll their children (this is especially helpful for postpartum mothers)

◆ Go to group therapy or join a support group

I am now leaving the house almost every day. Slowly and steadily, I have made the transition. You have to turn off the television and your electronics and get busy living. Building connections is an important key to recovery.

If one single aspect of SNAP gets out of balance, try to fix it right away. If you notice things are not going in the right direction, consider the tag and look at those things first.

I believed at one point in my life that I could be a hermit and heal. I now know that is not the truth. I have to be connected to other humans for my own sanity.

I incorporated this into my weekly goals. I speak about my mental health on a daily basis.

I am ending the silence. I don't want to hide anymore. I don't want to be embarrassed or ashamed, and I don't want to pretend that nothing is wrong. It might not be clear to a neighbor or clergy or family member that someone is in pain. But I have found my purpose, and I am delivering these messages to you for a reason. Please accept them. And check-in with those around you.

There is no one-size-fits-all solution to mental health. However, if we work as a team to advocate and share our experiences, the world will be a safer place. I intend to follow my dreams and promote unity for all of us. I became motivated by change. This new change was aligned with my intentions of a better life. My goal is to move forward everyday to increase my mental health balance.

When I am volunteering for a local LGBT group, I try to eat healthy, well-balanced meals and plan activities that are fun and exciting. I may get overwhelmed at certain busy times of the year, but I have learned that SNAP helps me regulate and balance myself.

Getting outside my comfort zone, I made myself visit people in need. I also ask people to go have coffee at the local coffee shop. We discuss life without using electronics.

Believe in your map and your compass. They will be your guides during times of stress and mind clutter. Of course, you should also know that I still fight my own battles.

Some days I fight with myself to get out of bed. I am still in recovery.

I recently battled a bad urinary infection and bronchitis. When I get sick, I feel isolated and withdrawn. However, I know it will soon pass and I will recuperate. As I improve my health, the days I feel "under the weather" are reduced. There are many steps to healing, and I still have some climbing to do. I am doing everything in my power to improve my well-being.

You must take action, even when you think there is no action to take.

It takes personal effort. Dig deep and remember that the creator of this universe is there by your side.

Now, I am able to take exciting trips with my family and friends. I attend concerts, have hobbies and collections, attend workshops and retreats. At long last, I have found my voice and am confident that neither me nor my story was a mistake.

During times of stress, any type of art and creating can really help. I've noticed that when I engage my creative side, my plan for healing started blooming.

My healing reminds me so much of summertime. It is like reading a good book under the warmth of the sun. The days are longer, and the nights are shorter. The summer season starts healing the earth from its cold, winter vulnerability.

There are so many exciting things I want to tell you. I want you to find purpose, too.

Focus on the positive aspects of your life. It does get better.

The tree of happiness made an imprint on my soul. That is what made me want to share my story.

Because of the tree, I look at things differently now. I see colors, see allies, hear birds, taste life, even smell victories ahead.

It feels like my passion has been restored during my healing process.

# Accepting

Disease does not define a person. Accepting your diagnosis is not fun, however, I believe this is the first step to wellness. Accepting your illness gives you permission to educate yourself, talk to others, and be part of your own treatment plan.

I am so much more than my disease. I am a mother, sister, friend, coach, spouse, grandmother, author, etc. I am not defined by my mental or physical health. I have chosen to live inside-out.

I spent so many years wondering why I was so different from everyone else, and perhaps you've felt the same.

Broken and wounded. Unwanted. Damaged. Not deserving forgiveness.

There was no relief. Old wounds kept reopening until they became infected. I avoided cleaning the dirt and grime, busying myself with just picking at the scabs.

The underlying hurt was based on a history of abuse. My core being was damaged. Child abuse can injure the brain and damage the spirit. We must understand the chain to break it.

I devoted many years to surviving the abuse. I felt alienated from others. I felt I didn't "belong" anywhere. These feeling negatively impacted my relationships with friends, family and romantic interests. I spent years in traditional therapy. Yes, it helped, but it was not enough.

I needed something else.

To thrive. To heal my distorted view of the world.

I regret that my own children were hurt during this time of recovery. I was not the parent I wanted to be or that they deserved. Recognizing this truth began my journey to victory. I claimed ownership and accountability and began to be the designer of my own life. I asked my children for forgiveness and I made many changes in my life to show them that I am putting actions behind my words.

Now I am asking, *what is my purpose? How do I get to my full potential?* You see this is my reflection now. I no longer dodge conversations about my past or original family. I join in with confidence. Now it seems I'm on fire. My soul is ignited with passion. I found my purpose: to share my story.

Accepting myself has been part of this journey. It did not happen overnight. If you think you will read this book and tomorrow you will be healed, you are wrong. The work is slow and continuous. I am still working on myself every day.

I know many of you are weathered having withstood much struggle. The battles have been fought for a cause and that is you. You have labored and are ready for change. I know this because you are reading this book.

Accept yourself here and now.

The war is not over it has just began. You too can share your story with someone. We must not abandon what we have been given. You are enough. You are not a mistake. Set yourself free.

◆◆◆◆

**Journaling Question:** How did this chapter make you feel?

_____

_____

_____

_____

_____

_____

_____

_____

_____

_____

_____

_____

_____

_____

_____

_____

## Following the Plan

The treatment plan can often change as a recipe for health however the main ingredients must always be consistent.

Follow your own version of the SNAP plan.

Following a treatment plan can be frustrating and you may see little growth at first. This is when you should use the networking support team around you.

The healing takes time. Be patient.

Take it slow and steady as in the turtle dream. It is time for you to recognize there is an abundance of joy out there for you. It will not come quickly or immediately. Take time and let the natural flow work for you. Too much can upset your balance. Slow down and let the healing begin. Be introspective. Let this help you become grounded with your feet planted firmly on the ground.

Reaching your potential is a collaborative process. Your team can help motivate you. If you have too many goals it might be overwhelming. So just prioritize and identify a few key goals on your plan. Remember your goals must be simple and measurable.

Example: *Cindy will manage her depression, by using the coping skills of SNAP. She will use the SNAP plan daily for three months. She will report to her therapist and support team.*

# Part 4 – The Impact

# Contributing

We can impact others by sharing our stories. I am not a speaker by nature but I have been asked to speak because of my story. Every day is an opportunity to share. Word-of-mouth takes place by sharing from one person to another. This is the time to enjoy the harvest of all your work. This is the most colorful season. Take time and build connections.

Just like sharing the dream about the turtle. People come up to me and want me to tell the story over and over again. Now the lesson of the turtle dream extends even further: When I had that dream, only three chapters of this book were written. That dream inspired and motivated me to create what you have in your hands today!

Once someone asked me who inspires me. I said the ordinary person doing extraordinary things.

A prime example is that in May of 2013, Oklahoma saw one of its most devastating disasters. A tornado hit an elementary school in Moore, Oklahoma. I was at a doctor's appointment just miles away. The whole hospital was rushed to the basement. We watched it live on television as the horror took place. I remember an article later about LaDonna Cobb, a mother going to pick up her daughters because of the impending bad weather. She stayed at the school to help save children's lives. This is what I find inspiring.

People of Oklahoma inspire me with their spirit.

A family named Dvorak in Perry, Oklahoma, about thirty five miles away from my hometown, were Family Farm of the Year. Farming plays a major role in human history. These roots go deep in the heartland. This ordinary rancher's life mirrors the words of Ecclesiastes, "There is a time to be born, a time to die, a time to plant, and a time to harvest."

I have a fear of public speaking. In this journey, I have had to face this fear head on. You see the road to happiness is not without fear. Since my book highlights fundamental strategies for creating a successful life people want to hear me speak about it. I started with just friends and family.

Speak it. Think it. Share it. Read it.

In December of 2014, I started a book club in my hometown. I hoped this would help me stay on track of my reading goals. I vowed to read twelve books a year. The group has been much more than a reading group. The fellowship and inspirational stories has been a blessing to my heart. You see everyone has a story. If you just take the time to listen, share, and be supportive. We have cried together, smiled together, laughed together and shared our dreams together. This journey has been more emotional than I ever thought it would be. Opening myself to others is fulfilling. I have met many wonderful people. It was so simple. I often ask myself why I didn't do this a long ago. The answer is that I was not ready.

Just a few months before I took my box of old writings out of the closet, I began to help deliver groceries to senior citizens in my community. This has been a very rewarding experience. I never knew so many seniors go hungry each month. Senior Citizens Centers all over America can use our help as we have many senior citizens in our community struggling to provide nutritious, life-sustaining meals for themselves. I have met some of the wisest and loving people during my deliveries. The weathered faces give a smile for a brown bag of groceries. It is all about impact. One of my favorite quotes is by Katrina Mayer: *At the end the day the only questions I ask myself are did I love enough? Did I laugh enough? Did I make a difference?*

People who can forgive inspire me. I resisted forgiveness for a long time.

Remember forgiveness is a decision, not an emotion. It offers grace instead of justice. Forgiveness opens up opportunities for the relationship to be restored. Forgiveness doesn't remove the wrongs. Forgiveness is power. There are many people in this world who inspire me because of their abilities to forgive.

Impact stories happen every day. In April of 2015, my adult sons, my spouse, and I went to Diamond Crater State Park in Arkansas for a retreat in an effort to reconnect with each other.

We had a great time at a cabin retreat. We met John. This is a letter I emailed him after our return home:

*Thank you for sharing your story about how God has touched your life. Also for the poem you read and the message you recited for me. I often tell people to be open to opportunities for healing. Our meeting was one of those opportunities. My tears were of joy and happiness as you delivered your message to me. I was touched with your courage. Friends and family often question how can I be so happy all the time? I've learned happiness is there the whole time within our reach: it's called God. He is our grace. Our only request is to surrender.*

*Let it go.*

*I have been doing a lot of thinking about why we chase happiness. We spend our whole lives doing so. This has come with lots of age and wisdom. My life has changed a lot over the last four years.*

*If someone had told me a year ago that getting fired from my job was going to start a new journey and provide the opportunity to refresh my life and reinvent myself, I would have protested, saying it would be too hard and that I wouldn't have the strength! Today, I see the beauty in this opportunity. My eyes are opened to more change, and I am grateful for lessons I've learned along the way! The strength is in the courage to take the first step on a not-so-familiar road! I want everyone to know every kind word is much appreciated! Every smile and brief "hello" never goes unnoticed. This is why we are all born, and this is why suffering and pain touches us. We then can have a chance to experience God's love.*

*I am simple person. I believe in random acts of kindness. When a new day unfolds before us, I will be prepared to impact someone. There is always an opportunity to complete what we were unable to do yesterday.*

*Thank you and have a great day!!*

My story was of value to others. I am sharing my dream with you right now as you read it, word by word.

Please pay it forward by making a difference to someone else today.

Enjoy this period of wellness filled with love, truth, connections, and gratitude.

# Networking

Networking has gone on almost as long as societies themselves have existed. It seems generation after generation, we keep redefining its meaning. It is such an important key to recovery. I thought it deserved its own chapter in this book.

Networking contributes to our roadmaps, building and engaging communities which will support us for a long time. So why can't it help you today, here and now?

Let me tell you of the power of networking in the Women's Suffrage Movement. It was important that Susan B. Anthony referenced that the right of citizens to vote shall not be abridged by the United Sates or by any state on the account of sex.

Two women in American History took the first steps of equality for all women. These women were Susan B. Anthony and Elizabeth Cady Stanton. One was a mother of seven children, and the other single with no children. They embarked on an adventure that was truly exceptional.

Both stepped out of their uncomfortable lives of powerlessness and devoted themselves to obtaining the right to vote for all women. This was their dream and their purpose.

This powerlessness ruptured a force of endless energy in this portrait of the sisterhood. The reservoir crumbled with the Women's Rights Convention in 1848 and the birth of desire in the midst of others with the same sex.

The Convention was like a child to most of these women.

They devoted themselves with the quality of rearing this child to be equal to all others. It took many decades of nurturing and commitment. Slow steady effort was the key to success.

Today, social media tools are more effective than email. How can we possibly realize the impact Facebook, You Tube, Twitter and the bloggers might have had on this injustice? The endless energy and the devotion could have been unparalleled. All women could have been connected to a sisterhood online.

There was a tipping point.

In this case in our history, these warriors could have given up on their dreams. They could have looked around at all their failures or felt like they did not deserve to win. But they did not. They continued to fight their fears and to battle onward. Slow and steady wins the race.

Here is one of my favorite quotes by Margaret Mead: *Never doubt that a small group of thoughtful, committed citizens can change the world. Indeed, it is the only thing that ever has.*

Let's go back to the story of women's right to vote and the impact of social networking with like-minded people. In 1872, Susan B. Anthony illegally cast her vote in the presidential election.

She delivered a speech in which she stated, "I stand here tonight for the alleged crime of having voted at the presidential election without having the right to vote."

Anthony quoted the preamble to the United States Constitution: "We, the People of the United States."

She asked the question regarding sex as a qualification of the right to vote.

This was Anthony's stand on her conviction of equality.

This is why it is such a great part of American history.

If all women knew of the fight for the right to vote and their suffrage, can you imagine the way history would have been written?

There would have been an upheaval.

They could have challenged the social order and achieved great things within months if the internet media tools were available to them during this time in history.

So how does all this tie into you? We must all find our tribes. People tend to live longer lives when they surround themselves with healthy behaviors and social relationships.

If we better understand ourselves and others, conflict will decrease. Healthier relationships inspire peace, forgiveness and new beginnings. They build value and worth.

We must advocate for each other.

We must share our stories and build connections. We must continue to challenge ourselves. We can raise awareness for others who are still struggling. We must remind ourselves to keep up-to-date on issues and to reach outside ourselves and discover there are people that need us.

If we get involved, we can make a big difference. Healing changes the universe.

We can inspire hope and help in others. We have to expose this invisible disease to others. Tell them we need to treat mental illness like every other chronic illness. We must invoke policy changes in our federal and local governments.

◆◆◆◆

**Journaling Questions:**

1. How can I make a difference?

   _____

   _____

   _____

   _____

   _____

   _____

2. Can early intervention help people that have mental illness?

   _____

   _____

   _____

   _____

   _____

3. How can I find community healthcare programs?

   _____

   _____

   _____

   _____

   _____

4. How can I integrate the health care system and mental illness?

_____

_____

_____

_____

_____

_____

5. How can I help end incarceration of individuals with serious mental health issues?

_____

_____

_____

_____

_____

_____

6. Do I feel segregated?

_____

_____

_____

_____

_____

_____

7. What is my experience in networking with others?

_____

_____

_____

_____

_____

_____

_____

# Gratitude

Developing an attitude of gratitude is an important skill to learn. We are all busy with jobs, children, traveling, and church. The hustle and bustle of life overwhelms many. Being grateful has power and happiness. Starting a journal was a significant step in my life. When writing in your journal, try to focus on the people and events for which you are grateful. Count each blessing. Don't limit the number of things you write.

Just write.

Take time and also think about your talents, abilities and service to others.

It is not always easy to be thankful, especially during times of stress and hardship. Seeing the sun through the clouds can be difficult. But try this belief. It's in these moments when gratitude is most needed.

We can be thankful for anything... jobs, school, scholarships, marriage, random acts of kindness, and even basic needs such as water, food and shelter.

I recently read an article about scientists from Berkeley who have begun to chart a course of research aimed at understanding gratitude and the circumstances in which it flourishes or diminishes. They're finding that people who practice gratitude consistently report a host of benefits:

◆ Stronger immune systems and lower blood pressure;

◆ Higher levels of positive emotions;

◆ More joy, optimism, and happiness;

◆ Acting with more generosity and compassion;

◆ Feeling less lonely and isolated.

◆◆◆◆

Here, I share some of my gratitude journal with you:

*May, 2004*

*My youngest child, Katelynn, is fifteen and going out tonight to the mall. I'm sure she will watching the "boys." She has grown into a beautiful fifteen-year-old girl. She acts sometimes like she hates hanging out with her family, but I know she craves it. We went to see Little Women at the Gaslight Theatre and she appeared engaged in the story. She is so smart and strong. I am so blessed. She is starting to be pulled by media, peers, school and other outside influences. It's like tug-of-war. I always thought my Katelynn would be a writer, or a star-gazer, but now it looks like she wants to be a fashion designer. Neither would bother me as a career for her. I am blessed to be around her while she grows to take on womanhood. I wonder if she knows that so long ago she kept me sane. She was very small when I was overwhelmed with my duffle bag of misery. She would lie next to me during spells of chronic depression. I thought "How can I give up with this small little girl looking in my eyes and touching my face?" I am grateful today and every day. I made the right choice to fight.*

As I reflect now on this journal entry, Katelynn is twenty-six. She is a great entrepreneur and a loving mother and wife.

*December, 2004*

*Today, I thought of my first born son, Tommy, Jr. (T.J). I developed some film, and his smiling face and sunny aura emerged from the photographs. He came for a visit last month from Pagosa Springs, Colorado. He has matured into an adult. I can hardly believe his is almost twenty-one. I truly enjoyed our visit. I miss his laughter and gentleness. I am full of gratitude for being a part of his journey. He often tells me I am his hero. I ponder parenthood often. Did I do a good job in raising my children? Did I give them enough love and kindness? Did I encourage them? I wish the divorce had not been so destructive. Neither love nor kindness was displayed by either party during the divorce. I regret that.*

My son is now thirty-one and a wonderful man.

*June, 2005*

*Barbara Stevison, Rhonda's mother, died today. Rhonda and I are truly blessed. The months and years of suffering have ended. My heart is heavy with sadness. Tears flow among all of her loved ones. I just hugged Rhonda tightly. Words of comfort were scarce. We began planning the funeral, flowers, songs, poems, and minister. It was a rush of moments in time to display someone's entire life. Today, someone I loved died. I am grateful Barbara was a part of my journey. She made a deep impact on my life. This is heartbreaking.*

◆◆◆◆

*August, 2005*

*My middle child Anita (Annie) got a pell grant to attend technology school. I believe this is good step forward towards freedom and gaining control over her life. She is starting to learn life is difficult. She is now twenty. Annie is very independent. She has a strong mind and sharp tongue. I believe she struggles right now. However, her time to bloom is coming in the near future. She often calls and tells me how much I mean to her, and we have been through a lot together. She said, "Mom, you never stopped loving me, and you've always supported me. I don't know where I would be today if you gave up on me." This is gratitude returned. I am grateful for a mother's love. I love all my children.*

As I ponder these thoughts today, Annie is a mother to four wonderful boys. She is still independent and strong-minded. She is on the local cub and boy scout committees. She is married and is a good friend.

◆◆◆◆

*June, 2010*

*I am one proud mom. Roy, my adopted son, graduated from Spartan college of Aeronautics. This guy has been through a ton of devastating moments in his life. He has overcome abandonment, the foster system, and mental health issues.*

*Today I am proud of his kindness, intelligence, and his free spirit. He is also generous and loves the outdoors. He offers to help whenever I need something, whether it's a hug or trimming my trees in the backyard. I have been honored to have this colorful character in my life.*

◆◆◆◆

*July, 2010*

*Rhonda and I started our goal to visit every state park in Oklahoma this summer. I am grateful to have the income to travel. I think these trips will counter my need to be alone. Sometimes we switch driver and navigator. This is very interesting. This makes you connect in different ways. The country is beautiful. We visited seven state parks this weekend and the Tahalequah area was impressive. I am grateful for God's Creation.*

I love my wife more and more each day.

◆◆◆◆

*March, 2014*

*The other day I had a visit from my sister Cheryl and her husband Craig. They often take time, driving two hours, to see me and help me fix things around the house. This time, Craig put in an oven. They have also helped put in a new handicapped toilet and railing, built me a shelf out of scraps in my garage, and even redone my bathroom to fix some plumbing issues.*

*When I was diagnosed with Sweet's Disease, I went from helping others to being the one on the receiving end of the gifts. I tried to return to work full-time, but after a while, my body just could not keep up with the stress so my doctor took me to part-time. Recently, at the end of 2013, my doctor took me off work completely. My savings have all been used for medical bills and medication. I filed for social security and was denied twice. My job of eight years terminated me in February. I tried to think that I could make it with the little bit of money that was coming in, however, I could not.*

*During our visit yesterday, my sister and brother-in-law asked if everything was okay. I tried to hold it together, but tears just came rolling down my face. They did not know I had been fired.*

*They told me all I had to do was ask, and that they would help me as much as they could. We hugged, and talked about what I needed help with. They looked over all my paperwork and helped me examine the reality. Then they had to run to the store to get some parts for the oven, and when they arrived back they handed me a wad of cash. They said, "This is our tithes, and we are cutting out the middleman. This is a gift, NOT A LOAN!" They also took my car and filled it up with gas. One spark of kindness and grace is all it takes and to help someone feeling so down. I've always had a giving heart and never really had to be on the receiving end. This gave me hope not because of the cash, but because I am so blessed to have friends and family who will help without me saying a word. We talked into the night about lifting people up and about what life really means when you take away all the material things. It really is about love. All kinds of love!! I am humble to see such compassion.*

◆◆◆◆

*April, 2014*

*I'm trying to journal more about my talents and abilities. I am searching for my purpose. I've be pondering it a lot lately. I feel the need to follow my dreams. I am at a strange age, with fifty right around the corner. I feel a need to make my life smaller and my group of friends and family tighter. Connections are all we really have in life. Too much of anything has always been my downfall. Now, I am thankful that I need only a few things and my love to keep me happy. I am using meditation daily. The more I meditate in silence, the more I let go of the things that do not serve me. I am grateful for meditation.*

◆◆◆◆

*July, 2014*

*It has been a while since my last entry. We celebrated the 4th of July at Katelynn's house. There was excitement, fun and smiles in every direction. The positive energy was endless. I visited with lots of people and felt relaxed and hopeful. For this I am grateful. Watching the sunset with people you love is amazing.*

◆◆◆◆

*April, 2015*

*I'm trying to journal more about my purpose. I've pondered it a lot lately. I feel the need to follow my dreams. I feel the need to reduce and to live smaller, not larger. My dream is a small cabin by the water. I want to watch the sun rise and set with my wife. I feel the need to connect with more people. I'm not sure how yet. The more I meditate, the more I feel the need to condense my life. In my most memorable moment of silence, I am not lonely. Let go. Forgive. Build anew. The sign of infinity refers to things without limits. I often see this sign in my meditations. I sent my mother a gift this week. I am not always a thoughtful or grateful daughter. I'm working on letting go of old negative energy and building a new more positive energy between us. She responded with a nice phone call.*

Thank you for letting me share my journal of gratitude with you.

**Suggested steps for starting a gratitude journal:**

1. Choose a journal or notebook.

2. Be consistent.

3. Write down inspirational quotes.

4. Elaborate on why you are thankful.

5. Don't wait for the right time.

6. Focus on people, not things.

7. Think of your talents.

8. Build your roadmap.

9. Fill the pages with knowledge.

10. Take a break from social media.

# Conclusion – Don't Give Up

No one wakes up one day wanting to be mentally ill. Try to look beyond your fears. Mental health issues are no different from other issues. The search for the right medication and treatment can take a long time.

It does get better.

As the goals are set and the achievements outweigh the failures, a sense of clarity and wisdom will began to evolve. You may not recognize it at first. It may be unfamiliar, but it is there.

Most people are broken and wounded. You are not alone.

Sometimes, we get stuck in a negative cycle of thoughts and actions that will prevent us from making progress.

Here is a quote from *The Alchemist* by Paulo Coelho: "We are told from childhood onward that everything we want to do is impossible. We grow up with this idea, and as the years accumulate, so too do the layers of prejudice, fear and guilt. There comes a time when our personal calling is so deeply buried in our soul as to be invisible. But it's still there."

There have been lots of times I wanted to give up. But my compass would not let me give up. I am a fighter. When I finally started learning my own coping skills, I was reborn. It was a daily process. It took lots of energy and effort. It took dedication and commitment.

Yes, I still have days that I struggle. I continue to fight, but this life is saved.

I have rediscovered my need for nature. I was on a trail, for the first time in over four years, in the foothills of Illinois late September. The fresh breeze enveloped me. I felt like the trees were whispering to me again, just as they had in my tree of happiness as a child. It was as if God was softly speaking to me, reminding me of the freedom I could have. When we got home, I found this Bible verse: (Job 33:4) *The Spirit of God has made me; the breath of the Almighty gives me life. Discover this freedom to choose happiness.*

I survived the worst part of my life, and this voice inside often reminds me of the tree of happiness. The way the tree held me up many years ago. The way the leaves whispered to me, and the warmth of the sun on my face. I often think, *am I good enough for God Almighty?*

The answer is always "YES!"

As I am writing this book, I know God's hands are an instrument of power, protection, provision, healing, guidance and comfort. Rhonda and I are joyfully joining a church. It is a new beginning for us. This is a celebration of faith. This is part of the Great Round for me. It is a coming home. I have struggled over the last thirty years with my higher power. My head resisted because people used the Bible as a weapon against me. My heart and soul always knew that I was loved by my head did not. I spent many years trying to connect my heart and head together. When I learned to let go of the past, I began the healing process. My journey to faith was rekindled. God moved through me to allow His rescue.

You must be able to accept what is, let go of what was, and have faith in what will be.

I often go back to the tree of happiness for comfort. The trunk held me up high on its branches as we constructed our tranquility. The wooden frame was nailed with hundreds of nails. Those nails were our struggles.

We were not alone, and neither are you.

Over and over I am reminded, *I am enough!*

I was forced to change my viewpoints, my fears, my relationships, my negative thoughts, my beliefs, and my suffering to find healing. When I started to transition I received life, freedom and happiness.

My purpose is here, right now. I'm holding nothing back.

The tree, a living thing that cares for itself, can also give you shade and shelter. You are God's creation. Hold on to the voice that will not let you quit! You will find your true potential and true happiness. You will be able to unload your duffle bag of pain.

I will close by reminding you that this is just the beginning. I never thought I could achieve this dream. At first, I wrestled with my fears of isolation and vulnerability. The internal work was a real challenge to me, too. I felt uncomfortable telling my story of recovery. I was brought to my knees several times during the writing of this book. I am still a work-in-process.

Then I reached for my own toolkit. I used the seven steps consistently. They worked. I learned to expand my awareness by stepping out of my own way. If an opportunity arose to try something different, I did not try to resist. I looked at the open space as a door to feel something new. It was my job to take a step forward as a human and as an author. There is an ending and beginning to everything. I must let go of my past regrets to make new choices, or I will get stuck in the things that no longer serve me. It takes lots of practice to develop one's self. I had to learn not to be a prisoner of the things I cannot change.

One of my favorite quotes by Helen Keller is *"When one door of happiness closes, another opens; but often we look so long at the closed door that we do not see the one which has been opened for us."*

The strength has always been inside you. Find a way to retrieve that strength. Recovery is possible. Healing is there.

Remember God, the sun, the tree and whispering leaves are for everyone.

Thank God for the tree of happiness.

## Afterward

Top Five Lessons from This Book:

1. Never give up on yourself.

2. Make a wellness/recovery plan.

3. Use SNAP: Sleep, Nutrition, Activity, and People.

4. Be empowered.

5. Make an impact.

Things I Learned Writing This Book:

1. Take a pause if necessary.

2. Be kind and tolerant.

3. Learn to say, "I'm sorry, please forgive me."

4. Listen to others.

5. Accept yourself just the way you are.

6. Find your natural rhythms and patterns.

7. Nurture your relationship with the Divine, whatever that means for you.

8. Ask for help when you need it.

9. Share your message with the world.

10. Never give up on your dreams.

# Sources and Notes

**Safe Cell:**

Nasar, Sylvia. *A Beautiful Mind: A Biography of John Forbes Nash, Jr., Winner of the Nobel Prize in Economics, (1994).* Published by Touchstone Books.

Grazer, B. (Producer), & Howard, R. (Director). *A Beautiful Mind* [Motion picture]. U.S.: Universal Pictures. (2001).

**Mental Evaluation:**

Alcohol, Drug Abuse, and Mental Health Administration. Report of the Secretary's Task Force on Youth Suicide. Volume 1: Overview and Recommendations. DHHS Pub. No. (ADM)89-1621. Washington, D.C.: Supt. of Does., U.S. Govt. Print. Off., 1989.

**Family Ties:**

Crisis Intervention Training (CIT). Dupont R, Cochran S, Pillsbury S. Crisis Intervention Team core elements. The University of Memphis School of Urban Affairs and Public Policy, Dept. of Criminology and Criminal Justice, CIT Center. Crisis Intervention Team website; 2007. Retrieved from http://cit.memphis.edu/CoreElements.pdf

Eleanor Roosevelt: It isn't enough to talk about peace. One must believe in it. And it isn't enough to believe in it. One must work at it. http://womenshistory.about.com/

Allison Krauss: Track: Where No one Stands Alone. Album: *I Know Who Holds Tomorrow*. 2010. https://www.amazon.com/

World Health Organization, Global Burden of Disease, 2004 Report: Colin Mathers, Ties Boerma and Doris Ma Fat. Bipolar disorder affects approximately 12.6 million individuals in the United States. http://www.who.int/healthinfo/

**The Journey:**

*The Road Less Traveled: A New Psychology of Love, Traditional Values and Spiritual Growth* (Simon & Schuster, 1978)

Human Rights Watch: Human Rights Watch team defends the rights of people worldwide. www.hrw.org

Mayor Frank Jackson, in Cleveland, Ohio. U.S. Attorney General
Eric Holder and the Justice Department:
http://www.cleveland.com/

**Surviving the 3 D's: Divorce, Death, and Disease:**
Depression & Divorce: http://www.webmd.com/
Sweet's Syndrome: http://www.ncbi.nlm.nih.gov/
Centers for Disease Control and Prevention (CDC):
http://www.cdc.gov/drugoverdose/
12-step programs: Alcoholics Anonymous (AA) (www.aa.org) A
twelve-step program is for people in recovery from alcohol
abuse.
Crnkovic, A. Elaine; DelCampo, Robert L. (March 1998). *"A
Systems Approach to the Treatment of Chemical Addiction."
Contemporary Family Therapy (Springer Science + Business
Media) 20 (1): 25–36. doi:10.1023/A:1025084516633*
Narcotics Anonymous (NA) is an addiction recovery organization
that was founded in 1953.

**Discharge:**
Corticosteroids: including cortisone, hydrocortisone and prednisone
— are useful in treating many conditions, such as rashes,
lupus and asthma. But these drugs also carry a risk of serious
side effects. http://www.mayoclinic.org/steroids/art-
20045692
Mother Teresa: (26 August 1910 – 5 September 1997) also known as
Blessed Teresa of Calcutta, MC, was an Albanian Roman
Catholic religious sister and missionary.
Chawla, Navin. *Mother Teresa: The Authorized Biography*. Diane
Pub Co. (March 1992). ISBN 978-0-7567-5548-5. First
published by Sinclair-Stevenson, UK

**Back to the Workforce:**
Family and Medical Leave Act: FMLA entitles eligible employees
of covered employers to take unpaid, job-protected leave for
specified family and medical reasons with continuation of
group health insurance coverage under the same terms and
conditions as if the employee had not taken leave.
http://www.dol.gov/whd/fmla/

Alice Morse Earle (April 27, 1851 – February 16, 1911) was an American historian and author from Worcester, Massachusetts.

**Trail of Tears:**
http://www.cherokee.org/AboutTheNation/History/TrailofTears/ABr iefHistoryoftheTrailofTears.aspx

**Education:**
http://tucollaborative.org/pdfs/Toolkits_Monographs_Guidebooks/re lationships_family_friends_intimacy/intimacy.pdf
Substance Abuse and Mental Health Services Administration (SAMHSA) www.samhsa.gov/
Farmer, Steven. *Healing words affirmations for adult children of Abusive Parents* http://www.amazon.com/

**Empowerment:**
Gilbert, Elizabeth. *Eat Pray Love.* http://www.amazon.com
Weight Watchers https://www.weightwatchers.com/us/
Alcoholics Anonymous http://www.aa.org/
Mohr, Tara. *Playing Big* http://www.amazon.com/
iempowerself.com Self empowerment is one of the simplest forms of taking charge of your life.
Walter M. Miller, Jr. You don't have a soul. You are a Soul. You have a body. *A Canticle for Leibowitz,* 1960.

**Impact:**
LaDonna Cobb http://www.nydailynews.com/news/national/
Dvorak in Perry, Oklahoma Family farm of the year http://www.crec.coop/
Mayer, Katrina. *The Mustard Seed* http://www.amazon.com/

**Networking:**
Women's Suffrage Movement: https://www.nwhm.org/online-exhibits/progressiveera/suffrage.html *and* http://www.nwhp.org/resources/womens-rights-movement/history-of-the-womens-rights-movement/

American anthropologist Margaret Mead (1901-78): Margaret Mead:
   *The Making of an American Icon* by Nancy C. Lutkehaus
   http://www.amazon.com/

**Gratitude:**
Expanding the science and practice of gratitude:
   http://greatergood.berkeley.edu/expandinggratitude

**Don't Give Up:**
The Alchemist by Paulo Coelho http://www.amazon.com/
Helen Keller: (June 27, 1880 – June 1, 1968) was an American
   author, political activist, and lecturer. She was the first deaf
   and blind person to earn a bachelor of arts degree.

# This is not the end, only the beginning.

### Congratulations!
You've invested in recovery by reading
this book to the end. Maybe it is your loved one, a co-worker, or
professional teammate who is struggling.
Help is here. Let the healing begin.
Process begins with a slow and steady pace.

### Check out our website:

# www.rootwordsalliance.com

for upcoming speaking engagements and book signings.
Our contact information and a media kit are on the website.

Imagine author, coach, entrepreneur Cynthia Stevison leading your
team through the transformational training process with customized
coaching over these seven steps.

### Let's Launch Together!
## Contact Cynthia today to begin the conversation.

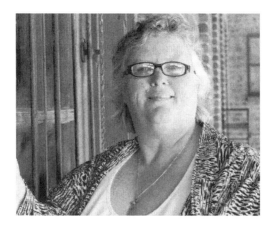

# Author. Coach. Speaker.

Made in the USA
Charleston, SC
09 April 2016